COPING SUCCESSFULLY WITH HAY FEVER

DR ROBERT YOUNGSON MB. ChB., DTM&H., DO., FRC Ophth, a former medical consultant is now a full-time writer. He is the author of eighteen popular medical and science books and has also written extensively on medical topics for *Reader's Digest* and *Good Housekeeping* books. He has made many radio broadcasts and has appeared on television.

Overcoming Common Problems Series

For a full list of titles please contact
Sheldon Press, Marylebone Road, London NW1 4DU

The Assertiveness Workbook
A plan for busy women
JOANNA GUTMANN

Birth Over Thirty
SHEILA KITZINGER

Body Language
How to read others' thoughts by their gestures
ALLAN PEASE

Body Language in Relationships
DAVID COHEN

Calm Down
How to cope with frustration and anger
DR PAUL HAUCK

Changing Course
How to take charge of your career
SUE DYSON AND STEPHEN HOARE

Comfort for Depression
JANET HORWOOD

Coping Successfully with Agoraphobia
DR KENNETH HAMBLY

Coping Successfully with Migraine
SUE DYSON

Coping Successfully with Pain
NEVILLE SHONE

Coping Successfully with Panic Attacks
SHIRLEY TRICKETT

Coping Successfully with Prostate Problems
ROSY REYNOLDS

Coping Successfully with Your Hyperactive Child
DR PAUL CARSON

Coping Successfully with Your Irritable Bowel
ROSEMARY NICOL

Coping Successfully with Your Second Child
FIONA MARSHALL

Coping with Anxiety and Depression
SHIRLEY TRICKETT

Coping with Blushing
DR ROBERT EDELMANN

Coping with Cot Death
SARAH MURPHY

Coping with Depression and Elation
DR PATRICK McKEON

Coping with Strokes
DR TOM SMITH

Coping with Suicide
DR DONALD SCOTT

Coping with Thrush
CAROLINE CLAYTON

Curing Arthritis Diet Book
MARGARET HILLS

Curing Arthritis – The Drug-Free Way
MARGARET HILLS

Curing Arthritis
More ways to a drug-free life
MARGARET HILLS

Curing Coughs, Colds and Flu – The Drug-Free Way
MARGARET HILLS

Curing Illness – The Drug-Free Way
MARGARET HILLS

Depression
DR PAUL HAUCK

Divorce and Separation
Every woman's guide to a new life
ANGELA WILLANS

Don't Blame Me!
How to stop blaming yourself and other people
TONY GOUGH

Everything You Need to Know about Shingles
DR ROBERT YOUNGSON

Family First Aid and Emergency Handbook
DR ANDREW STANWAY

Overcoming Common Problems Series

Fight Your Phobia and Win
DAVID LEWIS

Getting Along with People
DIANNE DOUBTFIRE

Getting Married
JOANNA MOORHEAD

Getting the Best for Your Bad Back
DR ANTHONY CAMPBELL

Goodbye Backache
DR DAVID IMRIE WITH COLLEEN DIMSON

Heart Attacks – Prevent and Survive
DR TOM SMITH

Helping Children Cope with Divorce
ROSEMARY WELLS

Helping Children Cope with Grief
ROSEMARY WELLS

Helping Children Cope with Stress
URSULA MARKHAM

Hold Your Head Up High
DR PAUL HAUCK

How to Be Your Own Best Friend
DR PAUL HAUCK

How to Cope with Splitting Up
VERA PEIFFER

How to Cope with Stress
DR PETER TYRER

How to Cope with Tinnitus and Hearing Loss
DR ROBERT YOUNGSON

How to Do What You Want to Do
DR PAUL HAUCK

How to Improve Your Confidence
DR KENNETH HAMBLY

How to Interview and Be Interviewed
MICHELE BROWN AND GYLES BRANDRETH

How to Love and Be Loved
DR PAUL HAUCK

How to Negotiate Successfully
PATRICK FORSYTH

How to Pass Your Driving Test
DONALD RIDLAND

How to Solve Your Problems
BRENDA ROGERS

How to Spot Your Child's Potential
CECILE DROUIN AND ALAIN DUBOS

How to Stand up for Yourself
DR PAUL HAUCK

How to Start a Conversation and Make Friends
DON GABOR

How to Stop Smoking
GEORGE TARGET

How to Stop Worrying
DR FRANK TALLIS

How to Survive Your Teenagers
SHEILA DAINOW

How to Untangle Your Emotional Knots
DR WINDY DRYDEN AND JACK GORDON

Hysterectomy
SUZIE HAYMAN

Is HRT Right for You?
DR ANNE MACGREGOR

The Incredible Sulk
DR WINDY DRYDEN

The Irritable Bowel Diet Book
ROSEMARY NICOL

The Irritable Bowel Stress Book
ROSEMARY NICOL

Jealousy
DR PAUL HAUCK

Learning from Experience
A woman's guide to getting older without panic
PATRICIA O'BRIEN

Learning to Live with Multiple Sclerosis
DR ROBERT POVEY, ROBIN DOWIE AND GILLIAN PRETT

Living Through Personal Crisis
ANN KAISER STEARNS

Living with Grief
DR TONY LAKE

Overcoming Common Problems Series

Living with High Blood Pressure
DR TOM SMITH

Loneliness
DR TONY LAKE

Making Marriage Work
DR PAUL HAUCK

Making the Most of Loving
GILL COX AND SHEILA DAINOW

Making the Most of Yourself
GILL COX AND SHEILA DAINOW

Making Time Work for You
An inner guide to time management
MAREK GITLIN

Managing Two Careers
PATRICIA O'BRIEN

Meeting People is Fun
DR PHYLLIS SHAW

Menopause
RAEWYN MACKENZIE

The Nervous Person's Companion
DR KENNETH HAMBLY

Overcoming Fears and Phobias
DR TONY WHITEHEAD

Overcoming Shyness
A woman's guide
DIANNE DOUBTFIRE

Overcoming Stress
DR VERNON COLEMAN

Overcoming Tension
DR KENNETH HAMBLY

Overcoming Your Nerves
DR TONY LAKE

The Parkinson's Disease Handbook
DR RICHARD GODWIN-AUSTEN

Say When!
Everything a woman needs to know about alcohol and drinking problems
ROSEMARY KENT

Self-defence for Everyday
Practical safety for women and men
PADDY O'BRIEN

Slay Your Own Dragons
How women can overcome self-sabotage in love and work
NANCY GOOD

Sleep Like a Dream – The Drug-Free Way
ROSEMARY NICOL

A Special Child in the Family
Living with your sick or disabled child
DIANA KIMPTON

Stop Smoking
BEN WICKS

Talking About Anorexia
How to cope with life without starving
MAROUSHKA MONRO

Talking About Miscarriage
SARAH MURPHY

Think Your Way to Happiness
DR WINDY DRYDEN AND JACK GORDON

Trying to Have a Baby?
Overcoming infertility and child loss
MAGGIE JONES

Understanding Obsessions and Compulsions
A self-help manual
DR FRANK TALLIS

Understanding Your Personality
Myers-Briggs and more
PATRICIA HEDGES

Vasectomy and Sterilization
Making the right decision
SUZIE HAYMAN

A Weight Off Your Mind
How to stop worrying about your body size
SUE DYSON

Why Be Afraid?
DR PAUL HAUCK

You and Your Varicose Veins
DR PATRICIA GILBERT

You Want Me to Do *What?*
A guide to persuasive communication
PATRICK FORSYTH

Overcoming Common Problems

COPING SUCCESSFULLY WITH HAY FEVER

Dr Robert Youngson

sheldon PRESS

First published in Great Britain in 1995 by
Sheldon Press, SPCK, Marylebone Road, London NW1 4DU

British Library Cataloguing-in-Publication Data
A catalogue record for this book is available from the British Library

ISBN 0–85969–720–7

Photoset by Deltatype Ltd, Ellesmere Port, Cheshire
Printed in Great Britain by Biddles Ltd, Guildford and King's Lynn

Contents

To Elaine

Introduction

Every year, millions of people – an estimated 20 per cent of the population – suffer distress, discomfort and embarrassment whenever the pollen count rises. Seasonal misery from hay fever, with itching and watering of eyes and noses, constant sneezing, nasal congestion and redness of the eyes, popping of the ears, constant clearing of the throat and coughing, takes much of the pleasure out of the best times of the year, and can prevent people from going to areas of natural beauty. It can also cause problems for young people taking important exams during the summer. Non-seasonal forms of the disorder affect people all the year round and these sometimes develop into more serious allergies. Some ten per cent of hay fever sufferers are also asthmatics or develop asthma.

Hay fever has been becoming increasingly common and is now ranked as the sixth most prevalent persistent condition in the major developed countries. In this respect it now outranks heart disease. Hay fever is not only unpleasant in its own right, but it also features a number of complications some of which can be even more troublesome – middle ear problems, hearing upsets, sinusitis, alteration of the sense of smell, sleep disturbances and mouth-breathing. Many conditions previously unsuspected of being allergic in nature are now known to be features of hay fever.

Recent years have seen great advances in the understanding of the immune system disturbances that underlie hay fever, and with these advances have come new and better forms of treatment. If you are a sufferer, the key to your personal management of hay fever is knowledge of these new facts. This book contains a straightforward account in clear, simple language of all the essential scientific facts underlying this annoying condition. It is not a medical textbook, but if you read it carefully the chances are that you will end up knowing more about hay fever than the average health professional. More importantly, you will know much that will help you to minimize the effect of this distressing condition on your life.

This book contains a number of 'case histories' illustrating important points in the story. It would not do to publish actual excerpts from clinical notes so these cases are presented in fictional form. All the events described in these cases, however, actually happened.

1
What is Hay Fever?

Although doctors commonly use the term *hay fever* when talking to patients, they don't use it so much among themselves. This is because doctors know that the condition has nothing to do with hay and doesn't cause fever. So the more formal members of the medical profession tend to stick to the medically correct term, seasonal allergic rhinitis (see p. 6). In this book, however, I can be as informal as I like, so I'm going to carry on using the well-known colourful term, however unscientific. First, a quick look at the background to the condition.

A short history of hay fever

The term 'hay fever' appears to have been used first in 1829 by a Dr Gordon writing in the now long-forgotten *Medical Gazette*. In his article on the condition he sometimes called it hay-asthma and sometimes hay-fever. There is another early reference in *Tweedie's System of Practical Medicine*, published in 1840. This early doctors' book talks of 'The summer catarrh, hay-fever or hay-asthma as it is termed from its supposed connexion with the effluvium of new hay.' In a letter written in 1840, the popular cleric and humorist Sydney Smith wrote: 'I am suffering from my old complaint hay-fever.' And in Martineau's *History of the Peace*, we find a reference, dated 1951, to another noted sufferer: 'The King enjoyed an exemption from his annual attack of hay-fever.'

Although these were the earliest uses of the term, the condition must have been well known to sufferers long before this. So far as we know, people have suffered from hay fever from the dawn of humankind. Certainly, as soon as people started taking an interest in the things that can go wrong with the body and writing down their observations and ideas, there have been accounts of the condition. Mostly it was referred to as 'catarrh' – a term applied to what we now know are several different conditions. One reference, of 1586, probably describing hay fever, goes: 'Sodainely choked with catarrhes which like to floods of waters, runne downewards.' In those days, the discharge from the nose and eyes was believed to come from the brain.

It was not until the 19th century that doctors began to get an idea of the real nature of hay fever. In 1819, a London physician, Dr John Bostock, wrote an account of a seasonal catarrhal condition affecting the nose. The description makes it clear that he was referring to hay fever. For a time, this condition was known as 'Bostock's summer catarrh'. The matter was taken a step further in 1831 when a detailed account of the condition was written by Dr John Elliotson. Elliotson's paper includes the perceptive remark by a patient that the disorder was brought on by pollen.

In 1872 and 1873 an English non-medical scientist, Charles Blackley, and an American scientist, Morril Wymann, who had been working independently on the problem for 20 years, published their results. Wymann noticed that hay fever symptoms were at their worst when ragweed flowered. He then sent parcels of ragweed to various people and produced the symptoms in those who were prone to hay fever. Blackley was a Manchester man and apprenticed to the printer and Quaker George Bradshaw of railway timetable fame. He was a hay fever sufferer and performed many experiments on himself and others to try to find the cause of the disorder. He applied pollens to many parts of his own body and even scratched some of it through the skin, causing a severe reaction. He also carried out experiments with sticky plates, some of them flown up in kites, to check for the presence of pollen in the atmosphere. Both his and Wymann's reports showed conclusively that hay fever was caused by grass and weed pollens. Another scientist was able to show that asthma could be caused in exactly the same way. These discoveries were of great interest to doctors who were, at the time, deeply concerned with the new ideas that many diseases were caused by invisible germs or microbes. This was a new idea

– a disorder caused by a substance that was not a germ and did not produce an infection that could be spread to others.

By the turn of the century those who knew most about the subject were aware that some people could be affected by certain substances in such a way that, although nothing happened at the first contact, they were somehow changed so that they became unusually sensitive to the substance. A second contact could then produce a severe reaction. In 1906 Dr Clemens Pirquet, working in Vienna, suggested that the new word 'allergy' should be applied to this mysterious hypersensitivity. This word quickly caught on.

At the same time, what at first seemed to be a completely different line of investigation was going on. This field of study had been started over a hundred years before by the English country doctor Edward Jenner who had found an effective preventive for the dreadful disease of smallpox. Jenner had heard a milkmaid say that she could never get smallpox because she had had the trivial condition of cowpox. She was simply repeating what was, to her, a well-known country belief. People who had contracted cowpox while milking never developed smallpox, even if they were in close contact with a case. So Jenner experimented on a boy, infecting him with material from a cowpox blister and then, rather rashly, infecting him with material from a severe case of smallpox. Both Jenner and the boy were lucky. The boy remained healthy, Jenner published his work, and the quiet country doctor became world famous. It was not long before thousands of people, including the Royal Family, had been vaccinated, and in recognition of his achievement, Parliament voted Jenner £30,000.

This was the beginning of the science of immunology. During the 19th century, many other protective inoculations were developed, especially by the French scientist Louis Pasteur and the German bacteriologist Robert Koch. At first, no one had the least idea how an attack of a disease could protect against another attack, but at the beginning of the 20th century the German bacteriologist Paul Ehrlich was able to prove that when the body was infected, it produced substances that combatted the infection. These substances remained in the body and, if a further infection occurred, were again produced, but in greater quantity so that there was complete protection.

Ehrlich won the Nobel Prize in medicine in 1908. By 1937, the nature of the protective substances were known. They were soluble proteins called *globulins*. From then on, progress was rapid. Hundreds of scientists devoted their lives to working out the processes of immunology and by 1962 everything important was known about antibodies.

You may be wondering what all this has to do with hay fever. The connection is quite simple. Hay fever is an allergy and allergy is the result of the immune system going slightly off the rails. So before you can understand hay fever you have to know a bit about the immune system and how it can go wrong. This is not really as complicated and difficult as you may think and it is well worth taking the trouble. These days, the immune system is very much in the news, and all well-informed people should know at least the basics of the subject. So, as well as helping you to cope with your hay fever, this book will enable you to understand other immune system disorders, such as AIDS. The real study of the scientific basis of hay fever starts in the next chapter, but first there are a few basic but important things to be said about the condition.

What is hay fever?

Strictly speaking, hay fever should be called *seasonal allergic rhinitis*. Another official terms is *pollenosis*. Both of these are a bit of a mouthful and neither seems likely to catch on with the general public, but they are worth explaining as they actually tell us a lot more than the term hay fever.

Rhinitis just means inflammation of the nose – in this case the inner lining of the nose. This word comes from Greek root *rhino*, which means 'nose' and the ending *-itis*, which means 'inflammation'. Every medical word ending in *-itis* is referring to inflammation of something. Appendicitis is inflammation of the appendix; gastritis is inflammation of the stomach; otitis, inflammation of the ear; dermatitis, inflammation of the skin; and so on. Rhinitis is not necessarily seasonal or allergic. Allergic rhinitis is nose lining inflammation caused by an allergy. You will learn all about allergy in the next chapter, and you may be surprised to find how interesting it is. If you are a hay fever sufferer, this is certainly something you should clearly understand.

A seasonal allergy, of course, is one occurring at a particular season of the year. This book is largely concerned with spring and summer allergic rhinitis – which are slightly different from each other – but it also deals with non-seasonal, or *perennial*, allergic rhinitis. Perennial just means 'occurring throughout the year'. This is due to many causes such as house dusts, house dust mites, or animal fur or skin flakes, and can affect sufferers at any time. This important form of the disorder is dealt with in Chapter 5. Here, we will concentrate on seasonal allergic rhinitis.

The word *pollenosis* sounds impressive, but it just means 'a condition related to pollen'. Doctors find the rather vague ending *-osis* quite useful, as it can be used to indicate any process, state, disease condition, cause or formation. If *-itis* doesn't fit, the chances are that *-osis* will. Pollenitis would hardly do, as that would mean inflammation of pollen – which is nonsense – so it has to be pollenosis. There are plenty of medical words ending in *-osis* – words like *fibrosis* (the development of fibrous tissue); *silicosis* (a lung disease caused by silicon dusts); *acidosis* (excess acid); *psychosis* (a disease of the mind); *agranulocytosis* (a shortage of white cells in the blood); and so on. The word pollenosis really doesn't tell us very much about the nature of the condition, however, so, having understood what it means, we can ignore it.

People with hay fever have developed an allergy to one or other of these pollens, spores, dusts, mite products or other animal products. Any object that causes an allergic response in a person is called an *allergen*. Contact between the allergen and the membranes lining the nose or eyes of the sensitized person results in an attack of hay fever.

You can read all about the symptoms of hay fever in Chapter 3.

It is hardly necessary to remind you of all the ways in which hay fever can interfere with your social, educational, business, professional or sexual life; if you were not concerned about this you would probably not be reading this book. But it is worth mentioning that, in Britain, up to 20 per cent of the population are affected to some degree by hay fever and some five per cent suffer significant interference with normal life and work.

Hay fever has been getting steadily more common over the whole course of the 20th century and there has been a striking increase in the incidence over the past 30 years. In Britain and America, hay fever accounts for about three per cent of all medical consultations, and a large number of sufferers never bother to consult their doctors. When allergic asthma, sinusitis and allergic skin reactions – the other diseases caused in the same way – are included, the figures are even more striking. In some countries, such as the United States, about a quarter of the population are affected. It is estimated that ten million Britons and 40 million Americans suffer from hay fever, asthma and other allergic diseases.

Pollens and other hay fever triggers

The spring type of seasonal allergy is triggered by airborne tree pollens, especially elm, birch, elder, plane, ash, pine, oak and maple. Most hay fever victims are allergic to grass pollens alone and suffer most severely a little later in the year. But some unfortunates are also allergic to tree and weed pollens, and have a bad time for months.

There are about 150 different species of grass in Britain but fortunately only about a dozen or so cause much trouble. If you are good at identifying grasses, you might be interested to know that among the common British grasses whose pollens cause hay fever are:

- Rye grass (*Lolium perenne*);
- Cocksfoot (*Dactylis glomerata*);
- Crested dog's tail (*Cynosurus cristatus*);

- Yorkshire fog grass (*Holcus lanatus*);
- Timothy grass (*Phleum pratense*).

Sometimes the problem is caused by airborne fungus spores, mainly of the genera *Aspergillus*, *Cladosporium* and *Alternaria*. You might be able to discover that you have an exclusive allergy to these if your attacks occur only at the times when they produce their spores. In Britain fungus spore production peaks in August and September. In other countries, check the situation in the late summer and early autumn (see also Chapter 11). These spores are usually released in a more localized geographic area than are tree or grass pollens. Weed pollens, such as those from the nettle dock or the water dock, can also cause hay fever. In North America, the big culprits are the green tassel-like flowers of the ragweed *Ambrosia artemisiitolia*.

The heavy, sticky pollen produced by brightly-coloured flowers is not a major source of trouble. This is not because such pollen cannot cause allergies – it can – but because this kind of pollen is not, to any great extent, carried by the wind. Flower pollen of this kind is transported by insects, especially bees, when it sticks to their legs and bodies.

The timing of hay fever

Different allergens cause their problems at different times of the year. The chances are that you will be affected by only one. Spring hay fever is triggered by tree pollens. Usually, oak tree pollen is the first to be released, followed by birch and plane tree pollen, then ash and pine. The summer type of allergy is due to grass and weed pollens. In the south of England, the worst time for grass pollen allergy is from mid-May until the end of July. North of Scotland sufferers have their worst time about five weeks later.

Pollen is released in the morning and rises throughout the afternoon. The grains are very small and light – only about 10–20 thousandths of a millimetre (10–20 microns) in diameter. This gives them a remarkable performance in air and they often rise to an altitude of about 3,000 metres (10,000 feet) In the country, pollen counts are usually highest between 3.30 and 6.00 pm. In town, the count rises to a peak at about 7.30 pm. The reason for the later timing in town is that, during the afternoons, rising thermal currents carry the pollen high out of harm's way. Unfortunately, during the evening, cooling of the air occurs and the pollen is brought down again.

A similar effect occurs at the seaside. Because of prevailing winds, much of the pollen is blown out to sea during the day. In the evening, however, winds tend to change and become onshore, bringing the pollen back in again. This is why sufferers at the seaside commonly have attacks during the evening.

The pollen count

Since pollen grains carried in the air are the trigger for attacks of hay fever, it is obviously of great interest to know how much pollen is in the lower atmosphere at any particular time. Pollen counting is of interest also to the meteorologists and is regularly done by them, as part of a more general measurement of atmospheric pollution.

Pollen counting is done by directing a continuous jet of the air being studied onto a stationary or moving surface specially prepared so that any pollen grains in the air will stick to it. The rate of flow of the air is known and the length of time the jet continues is accurately measured. In this way, the total volume of air involved is known. Sample areas of the surface are then counted by microscopy for adherent grains. This gives a measure of the concentration of pollen in the air.

Of course, the measurement really applies only to the area in which the measurement is done. Pollen levels can vary widely from place to place and official figures give only a general indication. They do, however, indicate that a risk is present. If the pollen count is high at the weather station where it is made, the chances are that it will be high elsewhere in the region.

Hay fever and the weather

The pollen count alone cannot fully predict whether you are in for trouble. If, however, pollen counts are taken in conjunction with the local weather situation, they can provide a much better forecast of the severity of the hay fever suffered by the population concerned. Given reliable weather forecasting, it is possible to predict the severity of hay fever to an accuracy as high as 80 per cent.

The worst kind of weather for hay fever is, unfortunately, the kind of weather most people enjoy best – no rain, plenty of sunshine and a rising temperature. In Holland, Dr F.T.M. Spieksma of Leiden University worked out a weather points system for hay fever sufferers. This gave a score of from 1 to 10. The lower the score the worse the weather and the better for hay fever victims. This score has been broadcast daily during the hay fever season on Dutch radio, giving sufferers the opportunity to adjust their treatment or modify their holiday plans.

In the lower atmosphere, the temperature is normally highest near the ground and becomes progressively cooler further up. Temperature inversion is the term given to a local situation in which the temperature is lower near the ground than at higher altitudes. The normal situation allows steady up-currents (*convection currents*) that carry up pollen and other pollutants, partly dispersing and diluting them. In a temperature inversion situation, however, convection current air flow cannot occur and the pollutants are kept down near the ground. Temperature inversion is very bad news for everyone, as it increases the concentration of all the undesirable material. It is the cause of the nasty smogs that can make so many cities uncomfortable and some, like Los Angeles, practically uninhabitable. It is particularly bad news for hay fever sufferers. Not only does it increase the pollen concentration, it also increases the other elements in the atmosphere that can make hay fever much worse.

The effect of other atmospheric pollutants

It has been known for a long time that hay fever is made worse by other pollutants in the atmosphere. The reason for this is gradually becoming clear. Many atmospheric pollutants, especially the nitrogen oxides from car exhausts and the ozone that is produced by the action of sunlight on these oxides, are damaging to the lining of the nose. Nature has provided us with a remarkable layer of lining cells to the respiratory system. These cells carry millions of fine, microscopic hair-like processes, called *cilia*, that beat backwards and forwards in a purposeful manner rather like wind blowing a field of ripe corn. This movement carries find particles and mucus out of the sensitive parts of the nose towards the nostrils.

Nitrogen oxides, even in quite low concentrations can damage the cilia-bearing cells. For instance, 0.4 parts per million of nitrogen dioxide will interfere with the action of the cilia. Two parts per million will kill the cilia cells. If this happens, pollen grains are obviously going to be kept longer in contact with the nose lining so that they are more likely to trigger an allergic response. The levels of these dangerous oxides from traffic fumes have been rising steadily for years and have been accompanied by a similar rise in the number and severity of cases of hay fever. This association also helps to explain the surprising fact that hay fever is commoner in towns than in the country in spite of the fact that pollens are more plentiful in the rural setting.

The outlook in hay fever

You may be encouraged to learn that hay fever disappears spontaneously in some five to ten per cent of sufferers. Why this should be remains a mystery. Those who are fortunate enough to enjoy this unexpected relief are people with comparatively mild seasonal allergy which has persisted for no more than about five years. Regrettably, if that period has passed and you are still prone to attacks, you are likely to be permanently affected. The only hope for a complete cure, in such a case, lies in the rather controversial desensitization treatment (see Chapter 7).

People with established hay fever or perennial allergic rhinitis (PAR) have about one chance in ten of developing the closely associated condition of allergic asthma. There is also a small chance of developing one or other of the various complications of hay fever (see Chapter 10). Don't be too discouraged by these gloomy prognostications. The chances are that you will have no such troubles. And there is a great deal you can do to control and alleviate the symptoms you do have.

Now that we have got the preliminaries out of the way, we can get down to the real business of understanding allergy. You may find the next chapter a little difficult, but it is really the most important chapter of the book and contains facts that should be known to every well-informed person. It is of particular importance to you if you are a hay fever sufferer, as it is only by understanding the scientific basis of the problem that you can tackle your problem logically and effectively.

2
Understanding Allergy

The term *allergy* is often used wrongly. Many substances can adversely affect the body and can do so in various ways, but these effects are not necessarily allergic. Unfortunately, the idea of allergy has caught the public imagination and some misunderstanding has resulted. Food allergy, for instance, is really quite rare, certainly far less common than is generally supposed. As for the 'total allergy syndrome', this is excessively rare – almost unknown – and much more likely to be a psychological problem than an allergy.

Allergy is an abnormal bodily response due to a minor defect in the action of the immune system of the body. This is not to say that the effects of this fault are necessarily minor – you would not be reading this book if they were. Sometimes these effects are very serious. But, as we shall see, much worse things can happen to the immune system than the defect that causes allergy. You will not be able to understand allergy without a basic knowledge of the immune system and how it works. So let's take a look at what is one of the most remarkable and interesting systems of the body.

Where is the immune system?

Don't be put off by the fact that this system – unlike the other systems of the body, such as the nervous system, the digestive system or the respiratory system – is largely invisible. This is because these other systems are based on large organs like the brain, the intestine and the lungs, while the immune system is based primarily on tiny, microscopic, individual and often free-roaming, cells. The whole body is, of course, made of cells but most of these are stuck together to form tissues and organs. The cells of the immune system are everywhere – in the blood, in the tissue fluids which bathe the body cells, and even between the cells that make up every organ of the body.

The only part of the immune system that you can actually see without a microscope are the collection of *lymph nodes* (usually called 'glands') and various masses of lymphoid tissue such as the tonsils, adenoids and spleen. The lymph nodes are small, soft, bean-shaped bodies found all over the body, but mainly in the neck, armpits, groins and around the main arteries of the chest and abdomen. These nodes are packed with immune system white cells, and are connected together by a fine network of clear tubes known as *lymphatics* which eventually drain into veins in the chest. The spleen is a larger, spongy organ lying in the upper left side of the abdomen, just to the left of the stomach. It has a very good blood supply and it, too, is packed with immune system cells.

How the immune system works

The object of the immune system is to keep the inside of our bodies free from living things like germs of all kinds, cancer cells and any abnormal and unwanted material that can cause damage. Without an effective immune system we are in real trouble, as people affected in some way by the AIDS epidemic know very well. Many of these invaders – viruses, bacteria, fungi and other single-celled parasites – damage local tissue and cause a reaction known as *inflammation*. The main feature of inflammation is a widening of the local blood vessels so that more blood than usual passes through the affected area. This is why an inflamed part looks red and feels hot. But this increase in blood supply serves a very useful purpose – it brings to the site of infection large numbers of the white blood cells that make up part of the immune system.

To do its job properly, the immune system has to be able to tell the difference between things that can be allowed to remain safely within the body and those that are dangerous or foreign and must be attacked. Any such foreign objects entering the body are called *antigens*. The immune system can immediately spot foreign antigens and attack them. In addition to dealing with foreign invaders, the immune system must also keep a constant watch over the body's own cells. If these are healthy, well and good. But if they have been attacked by viruses or have become cancerous, they must be destroyed. Without this constant surveillance for cells with cancerous changes, we would all have been dead long ago. Unfortunately, there is a limit to the efficiency of the immune system and, sometimes, too many cells with these changes occur for the system to deal with. In that event an established cancer develops.

The antibodies

The job of identifying foreign material is performed by certain phagocytes, known as *macrophages*. When a macrophage engulfs a foreign organism or cell it immediately alerts other cells of the immune system. These cells are called *lymphocytes* and there are two main kinds – the T lymphocytes and the B lymphocytes. These cells are so important, and have to be mentioned so often by people concerned with the immune system, that they are usually referred to simply as 'T cells' and 'B cells'. But you should remember that they are all lymphocytes.

T cells pick up information from macrophages. The B cells have a different job. Their function is to produce certain protein substances called *antibodies*. Each B cell can produce only one kind of antibody. But there are literally thousands of different kinds of B cells, each capable of making a different antibody best suited to deal with a particular kind of foreign invader.

After the macrophages and their attendant T cells have completed the recognition process, an extraordinary thing happens. The T cells look over the range of the B lymphocytes to find the one capable of producing the most effective antibody against the invader. When they find it, they instruct this cell to multiply and produce numerous daughter lymphocytes, all identical to the one that started. A population of identical cells is called a *clone*. This clone of B cells now starts to produce large quantities of antibodies. Each one may synthesize 2,000 antibodies per minute, and the clone may contain millions of B cells. The antibodies are Y-shaped proteins that quickly bind on to and inactivate the antigens. Once this has occurred, these foreign objects and infected or diseased body cells fall easy prey to other phagocytes and are soon eaten up and destroyed.

B lymphocytes that have been activated in this way can survive for many years, preventing us from suffering a second attack of many infectious diseases. When a second infection occurs, they are ready and waiting, and will, if necessary, clone more copies of themselves to produce more of the same antibody. This is also how immunization works. It is a fairly easy matter to identify antibodies precisely from a small sample of blood. Different people who have had the same infection carry the same antibodies and these can be pinpointed in the laboratory. So it is easy to tell whether a person has had any particular infection, even if they have been cured of it years before.

More about antibodies

Antibodies are proteins. Some proteins, such as those of meat (muscle), are fairly obvious; others are not because they are dissolved in the blood. The soluble proteins include a group called the globulins and these include all the antibodies. Because these globulins are concerned with the immune system, they are called *immunoglobulins*. Although the body can produce many thousands of different antibodies, these fall into five well-defined groups. The name immunoglobulin is already rather a mouthful and, since it is often necessary to say which group you are concerned with, it is a good idea to shorten the name. Doctors therefore talk of *Ig* for immunoglobulin and then add the letter that indicates the group.

The most plentiful group of antibodies is immunoglobulin class G, usually abbreviated to *IgG* or often called *gamma globulin*. Three quarters of the immunoglobulins in the blood of healthy people are IgG. IgG antibodies are concerned with protection against a wide range of germs. Only one of the other four antibody groups need concern us here – the immunoglobulin class E. IgE is the antibody type that is involved in hay fever. It is also the antibody group concerned in causing asthma and other allergic reactions. Needless to say, you will find quite a lot about IgE in this book. Like all the other immunoglobulins, IgE is produced by B cells. These are present in large numbers in the nose lining, the tonsils and in the wall of the intestine.

People who do not have allergy problems produce hardly any IgE; people with hay fever, allergic asthma, severe allergies and eczema have lots of it. You can even cause an entirely healthy person to develop hay fever simply by giving him or her an injection of the serum from a hay fever sufferer. This serum contains IgE and by giving this immunoglobulin you can convert a non-allergic person into an allergic person.

Recent research has shown that the body can manufacture IgE only if certain types of T cells of the immune system are present. These cells, the 'helper' T cells are, incidentally, the ones that get knocked out by the human immunodeficiency virus (HIV), thus causing AIDS. It seems likely that people who do not suffer from hay fever have very few of this particular group of helper T cells, whereas those who do have plenty of them.

In spite of a great deal of research, we still don't know for certain what IgE is for. The function of all the other immunoglobulin groups is clear and they are all obviously beneficial, but IgE seems to be good for nothing and when it does have an effect, that effect is harmful. There was thus great excitement among the immunologists a few years ago when it was found that people in the tropics with worm parasites had high levels of IgE in their bodies. This suggested that the original function of IgE might have been to protect against such parasites. Presumably, worms and other similar parasites are no more enthusiastic about the effects of IgE than people are. Be that as it may, the idea provides cold comfort to people who are never likely to have a problem with worms but who greet the spring of each year with sinking hearts.

How can the immune system go wrong?

This can happen in various ways. Because of AIDS, the best known, these days, is immune deficiency. This group of diseases had, however, been familiar to doctors for many years before AIDS appeared. Immune deficiency can be present at birth as a genetic disorder of various degrees of severity. In rare cases this is so complete that the baby has to be kept in a sealed chamber if there is to be any chance of surviving. Immune deficiency can also be acquired later in life in various ways. These include:

- insufficient protein intake from malnutrition to make antibodies;
- loss of antibodies in the urine as a result of kidney disease;
- radiation damage affecting the production of immune system cells;
- long-term use of antibiotics and other drugs that damage the immune system;
- the effect of old age;
- the acquired immune deficiency syndrome (AIDS).

AIDS is caused by HIV, which attacks T cells, preventing them from carrying out their normal task of identifying foreign invaders. As a result, the body becomes prone to develop infections of all kinds and is much more liable to develop cancer.

So what has all this to do with allergy?

You may be wondering why it is that, although all of us breathe in pollen grains from the atmosphere, only some of us get hay fever. The reason is that there is a genetic condition called *atopy* that causes people to react to certain substances in a certain way. Atopy is hereditary and may show itself either as hay fever or as asthma or as the skin problem *eczema*. Some unfortunates have all three but usually one or other predominates.

People who get hay fever have an inherited tendency to become over-sensitive to substances, specifically certain proteins present in pollen grains, that are completely harmless to 80 per cent of the population. These substances are commonly called *allergens*. You already know quite a number of other important things about them, but to recapitulate briefly, these are that:

- they are *antigens*;
- the body recognizes them as foreign;
- the body reacts to them by producing antibodies;
- these antibodies are proteins, known as immunoglobulins;
- they are produced by B lymphocytes;
- the antibodies produced are in a special immunoglobulins class known as class E;
- they are therefore known as IgE.

In hay fever the antigens are in the seasonal pollens in the inhaled air. These pollen grains enter the nose and are trapped by a layer of sticky mucus. The fine moving hairs (cilia) on the lining cells immediately start to try to move them out. But before they can get rid of them, a chemical activator (*enzyme*) called *lysozyme*, that is present in the tissues, digests off the outer coats of the grains and releases the protein antigens.

Now we come to the villains of the piece.

The mast cells

Back in 1877 the brilliant German scientist Paul Ehrlich – the first man to produce an effective antibacterial drug that could be taken internally – noticed some rather peculiar cells under his microscope and took the trouble to record his observations. These cells, when stained, were seen to be packed with round bodies like granules. Enrlich assumed that these cells were phagocytes and that the granules were 'food' particles that the cells had taken up. For this reason he decided to call it them mast cells. (In German, the word *mast* means 'a feed for fattening'.) Neither Ehrlich nor anyone else had any idea what the mast cells did, so after that they were largely forgotten. Today, the mast cells are at the centre of interest of anyone concerned with allergies and especially hay fever.

Situated within and just under the lining of the nose in people who suffer from hay fever, allergic asthma and severe allergies, are millions of mast cells. These are formed in the bone marrow and are carried in the blood to all parts of the body where they lodge in most kinds of tissue. Interestingly, people who do not suffer from hay fever have comparatively few mast cells in their nose linings.

Mast cells can easily be seen with a modern microscope. If a swab or a scraping containing mast cells is stained in the usual manner for microscopy, these cells are seen to be full of tiny, deep-staining spots known as granules. These granule-filled mast cells are of basic importance in allergy. In people with hay fever the number of mast cells in the nose and throat lining increases steadily as the hay fever season advances.

The granules in the mast cells are actually tiny droplets containing a very nasty mixture of highly active substances. These substances have various effects, all of them unpleasant. The most important and best known of them is called *histamine* and this is the one you should know about. Histamine does no harm so long as it remains safely locked up in the granules of the mast cells. But if these granules are released it is free to act.

This is what histamine does:

- it causes the secreting cells in the nose lining to produce mucus and watery secretions;
- it increases the leakage of fluid from small veins so that membranes swell;
- it attacks local nerve endings causing itching and burning;
- it contracts smooth muscles, including those in the walls of the air tubes (bronchioles) of the lungs.

In addition to histamine, freed granules release protein-splitting enzymes, called *proteases*, which can damage small blood vessels. They also release substances called prostaglandins that are powerful nerve stimulators and a range of substances called *leukotrienes*, which are even more potent narrowers of the air tubes than histamine. All this, of course, leads to the general misery of the hay fever victim. This, too, is the mechanism that leads to allergic asthma.

There is another important point to be made about mast cells. If the amount of natural body steroid – the secretion of the adrenal glands situated on top of the kidneys – is increased, mast cells are seriously discouraged from appearing. As we shall see, this fact can be exploited as a way of preventing, or minimizing the severity of, hay fever.

Degranulation

The central fact to appreciate about mast cells is that they love IgE. Mast cells have thousands of special sites on their surfaces that IgE antibodies fit into perfectly. These are called IgE receptor sites. So anyone who produces a lot of the particular type of IgE produced by hay fever victims is going to have mast cells already covered with IgE. This is when another remarkable thing happens.

You already know that antibodies work by latching onto antigens. This is their whole function in life. They are, chemically, of just the right shape to fit the antigens like a key fits a lock. When IgE is in place on the mast cells and new pollen antigens come along, the latter, of course, immediately get linked to the IgE. But this happens in a rather peculiar way. Instead of one antigen attaching to one antibody, each pollen antigen bridges across two or more adjacent IgE antibodies. This causes the outer membrane of the mast cell to distort so severely that it ruptures. And, of course, when that happens, the granules pour out. This is called *degranulation*.

Degranulation occurs within 20 minutes of exposure to the pollen antigen and it occurs even in mast cells one millimetre below the surface. Degranulation, of course, releases histamine and all the other unpleasant substances that act on the local tissues to cause the symptoms of hay fever.

Late effects

Unfortunately, this is not necessarily all that happens. For many people, hay fever is not much more than a considerable nuisance. But for others various complications may arise, and some are quite serious. You can read about them in Chapter 10. The longer you have hay fever, the more severe it tends to become. The levels of IgE rise progressively and the number of mast cells in your upper respiratory tract increases. The sensitivity to the allergen also increases so that repeated contact produces an increased release of histamine. Perhaps worst of all is the possibility that this process may lead, eventually, to permanent changes in the nose and surrounding areas, in the ears or even in the lungs. Doctors are still arguing about whether or not this latter misfortune actually occurs.

Is hay fever hereditary?

Many cases certainly are hereditary. These are hay fever sufferers with a family history of other allergic problems such as asthma, eczema, nettle-rash, severe reactions to bee and other stings (*anaphylaxis*) and sometimes food allergy. As we have seen, this tendency is called *atopy*, and such people produce far larger quantities of IgE antibodies than do non-allergic people.

Families with atopy have been studied to see whether the genetic basis of allergy can be clarified. Recent research at the Churchill Hospital, Oxford has shown that it can. The scientists there located the gene responsible for producing the receptor sites on the mast cells to which the IgE molecules attach themselves. In June 1994 they revealed that many families with atopy have a particular variant (*mutation*) of the IgE receptor gene. Surprisingly, this abnormal gene has, in every case, been found to be inherited from the mother. The IgE receptor sites produced by this gene are only very slightly different from those on the mast cells of people without atopy. But this slight difference is enough to affect the way mast cells with IgE respond to pollen grains. It seems that the abnormal IgE receptor sites simply make the mast cells much more sensitive to the triggering effect of the pollen grains.

You will be relieved to know that we are now through the hard part and that from now on it's all pretty plain sailing. There is just one last bit of preliminary study before we go on to deal with the symptoms of hay fever.

More about the nose

Although hay fever involves parts other than the nose, this is the region that suffers the most sustained attack. So, as a hay fever sufferer, the more you know about your nose the better. You have already learned about the remarkable cilia that waft out foreign material caught by the mucus (see Chapter 1). But there is good deal more to the nose than that.

The shape of the nose is determined by a short bone that protrudes from the lower part of the forehead – the nasal bone – and a number of cartilages that are connected together by fibrous tissue. The two halves of the nose are separated by a thin partition made of cartilage in front and bone behind. This is called the *nasal septum*. It is quite easy to change the shape of a nose by sculpting away at the cartilages and to change the degree of protrusion of the nose by filing away part of the bone. The bone and cartilage is covered externally with skin and internally with a layer of mucous membrane. The inner parts of three of the cartilages on each side are curled up so as to increase the surface area over which the inhaled air must pass. These curly, mucous membrane-covered plates are called *turbinates*.

The nose has a remarkably good blood supply – a fact reflected in the ease with which it can be made to bleed. The lining of the nose and the zone between the lining and the cartilages and bone contain many blood vessels – both arteries and veins. The curled turbinates and the septum carry quite large vein channels that can swell easily when filled with blood. For this reason these are called *pseudo-erectile tissue*. The condition popularly known as 'stuffy nose' is due to the swelling of these veins and the general congestion of the mucous membrane. Vein channel erection is under the control of part of the nervous system (the *autonomic* system) and, even in perfect health, this usually causes alternate swelling of one side and then the other. This alternation occurs at intervals of between two and seven hours. It is, or course, much more obvious when you have a cold or are suffering from hay fever.

This rich blood supply is capable of raising the temperature of the inspired air by as much as 25°C as it passes from the atmosphere to the back of the nose. The inner openings of the nasal passages are the narrowest part of the entire respiratory system and as a result it is quite hard to get enough air through the nose when the body's oxygen requirements are raised by strong exertion. When the requirement rises above about 30 litres per minute we are forced to open our mouths.

The lining mucous membrane is exceptional in its ability to produce watery secretion and mucus. The water production can be turned on like a tap. This is because of the profusion of glands in the mucous membrane. In the nose there are eight times as many secreting glands in each square millimetre than in the rest of the respiratory system. People who suffer from hay fever know all about the remarkable power of the nose to produce these secretions.

3
The Symptoms of Hay Fever

Hay fever is not so much a disease as a collection of symptoms. If you take away the symptoms there is really not much left that can harm you. So, however unpleasant, distressing or temporarily disabling the symptoms, hay fever, in itself, is not a dangerous condition. Since symptoms are such an important part of the disorder, let's take a closer look at them.

Sneezing and itching

The most obvious and common symptom of hay fever is sneezing. Millions of people who suffer mildly from hay fever have no more trouble from it than occasional sneezing. At worst they have a succession of uncontrollable sneezes. Sneezing, of course, is a response to irritation occurring within the nose. Its function is to get rid of any irritant or potentially damaging material that finds its way into the nose, especially particles of matter that might be inhaled. The sneezing is not caused directly by the pollen grains; these are much too small to do so. It is caused by histamine (see chapter 2), released by the mast cells, and acting directly on nerve endings lying between the cells of the lining membrane of the nose.

When these nerve receptors are stimulated by the histamine, several things happen. First there is an immediate reflex indrawing of a very deep breath. Then the vocal cords in the *larynx* (voice box) are pressed tightly together. Next, the muscles of the chest and the diaphragm tighten sharply so as to compress the air in the lungs. At the same time, the tongue is pressed tightly against the roof of the mouth and the soft palate moved clear to open the way to the nose. Finally, the vocal cords are suddenly pulled apart so that a blast of air rushes up the windpipe and out through the nose. This is a very efficient way of getting rid of fluff or other foreign material. Unfortunately, in the case of hay fever, the only things worth getting rid of – the pollen grains – have already done their harm, so the sneeze serves no useful purpose.

Sneezing is nearly always associated with itching and this may be severe. In children, this persistent itching causes the child repeatedly to rub the nose upwards to try to relieve it. This may happen so often that the child develops an obvious transverse ridge or crease across the skin of the lower part of the nose. This sign is well known to specialists in the subject and is known as the 'allergic salute'.

Fluid and mucus production

Another distressing and embarrassing feature of hay fever is the watery and mucus discharge. Like other cavities, passages and hollow internal organs of the body the nose is lined with a surface called a mucous membrane. Mucous membrane also lines the inner surfaces of the eyelids and covers the whites of the eyes. In the latter location, the mucous membrane is called the *conjunctiva*. Mucous membranes contain large numbers of goblet-shaped cells, which are actually individual secreting glands, and other small fluid-secreting glands. These normally produce moderate quantities of a watery fluid, to keep the membrane moist, and mucus to keep the surface sticky and trap foreign material. Mucus is a slimy, jelly-like material, chemically known as a *mucopolysaccharide* or *glycoprotein*. It has essential protective and lubricating properties and life would be unpleasant, and perhaps impossible, without it. In the nose, the main function of mucus is to assist in the conditioning of inhaled air and to provide a sticky coating that traps inhaled material.

In hay fever, the histamine and other substances released when the mast cells degranulate are powerfully irritating to the mucous membranes of the nose and eyes. The membranes of the eyes contain large numbers of tiny accessory tear glands and fewer mucus glands. As a result of histamine release, all the glands of the membranes start to work overtime, secreting fluid and mucus, sometimes, seemingly, to the limit of their ability.

Again, this excessive secretion serves no useful purpose except, possibly, to dilute the histamine. It can, however, cause severe distress to the sufferer. Running nose and eyes can be temporarily disabling as well as embarrassing and can, occasionally, be dangerously distracting. It doesn't help your driving concentration, for instance.

Nasal congestion

As well as causing overactivity of the secretory glands in the nose and eyes, the effects of histamine are to cause swelling of all the cells of the mucous membrane. In addition, the blood vessels of the mucous membrane and those in the network below it widen, pushing the swollen mucous membrane further away from the underlying cartilages. The resulting swelling can be so severe as to obstruct the nose completely. The increased blood supply also means that increased amounts of watery fluid leak out from these blood vessels to add to the swelling of the membrane. An increase in the blood supply also promotes more rapid secretion of the gland cells. If the nose is blocked, secretions may drip down from the rear openings of the nostrils into the throat. This is called *post-nasal drip*.

Persistent inflammation of this kind actually causes the mucous membrane of the nose to become more sensitive to mast cell granule products. It also increases the sensitivity to other irritants that have nothing to do with pollen or the allergic response. People with hay fever are more sensitive to atmospheric pollution than other people and, as we have seen, some atmospheric pollutants interfere with the ciliary action of the nose lining (see Chapter 1) thus prolonging the action of pollen. Persistence of the symptoms of hay fever after the pollen season may be due to this increase in general sensitivity of the nasal mucous membrane. This is one of the causes of perennial allergic rhinitis.

Nasal obstruction from swelling of the mucous membranes forces the affected person to mouth-breathe and affects the quality of the voice. It can also have a serious effect on the functioning of the mucous-membrane-lined *eustachian tubes* that run from the back of the nose to the cavities of the middle ears. These tubes need to be intermittently open so that the pressure can be equalized on both sides of each ear drum. Eustachian blockage from mucous membrane swelling causes deafness and an unpleasant sense of fullness in the head. Many cases of intermittent eustachian catarrh are caused by allergic swelling of the mucous membrane. Long-term blockage can even lead to infection of the middle ear (*otitis media*). This can do permanent harm (see Chapter 10).

In the case of the nose, only the sufferer is much aware of what is happening. In the case of the eyes, however, the effect is highly conspicuous and sometimes almost alarming to the observer.

Eye symptoms

Irritated mucous membranes become inflamed and red and this is readily visible in the eyes of a victim. Even more striking is oedema of the conjunctivas, which may balloon out between the lids as if they were inflated. The conjunctivas are firmly fixed around the margins of the corneas and are securely attached to the insides of the lids. But over the whites of the eyes they lie loosely on the globes. It is thus possible for considerable quantities of fluid to collect *underneath* the conjunctiva causing the dramatic appearance. Sometimes this conjunctival oedema is so severe that the corneas appear as round discs at the bottom of a gelatinous pit and the eyelids are unable to close over the swollen membrane. Fortunately, this kind of oedema always settles.

Another striking effect of allergy on the conjunctivas is known as *vernal catarrh* or *vernal conjunctivitis*. This condition is rare in temperate climates but is very common in tropical and sub-tropical areas and in the Middle East. In such regions it affects mainly children, boys much more often than girls. In vernal catarrh, the conjunctivas become persistently thickened so that a raised, tyre-shaped, gelatinous ring of permanently swollen conjunctiva forms around each cornea. There is intolerable itching, causing great distress, and a stringy, tenacious discharge from the eyes. Vernal conjunctivitis can also cause gelatinous swellings (like cooked sago grains) to develop on the inner surface of the upper lids, with considerable swelling of the lids and severe itching and discharge. In both of these conditions the conjunctivas are packed with mast cells.

Other symptoms

Hay fever sufferers often experience quite strong itching of the ears, itching that may make scratching irresistible. This is not a histamine effect, however, but a referred sensation due to the fact that the same nerve that provides sensation to the back of the throat also supplies the ear canal and the outer ear. Stimulation of the throat branches of this nerve by histamine and other mast cell granule products can cause a sensation to be passed to the ears.

There is another, and more important, way in which hay fever can affect the ears. The swelling of the mucous membrane at the back of the nose and throat can cause a temporary blockage of one or both of the eustachian tubes. These must be capable of passing air if the ears are to work properly. Any obstruction of the tubes causes an uncomfortable feeling of fullness in the ears and sometimes a degree of deafness or a change in the quality of the hearing. You can read more about this in the chapter on complications (Chapter 10).

It is not widely appreciated that many coughs are caused by the same allergic process that causes hay fever. If you find yourself with an intermittent dry cough that seems to come on for no reason in the spring or summer and then disappears as suddenly as it came, there is a distant possibility that this could be the cause. Most of the allergens that cause hay fever are large enough to be trapped in the nose; some, however, are smaller and are able to get down into the air tubes of the lungs.

Secondary symptoms

The symptoms described above are those caused directly by the immunological process. But anyone affected, to any serious extent, by these symptoms will inevitably have a psychological reaction to them. These reactive psychological symptoms are important and a chapter has been devoted to them. You can read about the emotional dimension in Chapter 8.

4

How Hay Fever is Diagnosed

Hay fever is a condition you can probably diagnose for yourself with a good deal of certainty. But the matter is not always so easy as you might think. In typical and well-marked cases of hay fever the diagnosis is obvious. Here is a review of the symptoms:

- itching and pricking of the nose, palate, throat and eyes;
- paroxysms of sneezing;
- runny nose and eyes;
- stuffiness of the nose with partial or total blockage;
- irritability;
- depression;
- tiredness;
- a general feeling of being unwell (*malaise*).

If these symptoms are associated with exposure to pollen at the appropriate time of the year, there can be little doubt about the diagnosis. Not all cases, however, are so typical and few show all the features just listed. In fact, the great majority of cases of hay fever are very mild, and many are not recognized for what they are. Millions of people sneeze frequently during the pollen seasons but have no other symptoms and are unaware that they have hay fever.

Another important indication that the trouble is hay fever is the fact that the symptoms are worse at certain times of the day than at others. This occurs in hay fever because of differences in the amount of pollen in the atmosphere (see Chapter 1).

Finally, you must try to distinguish hay fever – which is seasonal, from perennial allergic rhinitis (PAR) – which occurs all the year round. The two conditions are otherwise identical, although caused by different allergens. Both involve IgE and mast cells. If the allergy is perennial, you have to consider the possible causes.

Clinical diagnosis

Not all cases of hay fever are as easy to diagnose as the above account suggests. In some, the cause is less obvious and some present in an unusual way. Such cases really require medical attention. Sometimes, in spite of taking a careful history and enquiring into all the obvious possibilities for allergy, the doctor may still be uncertain about the diagnosis. Here is a case history in which this happened.

Introduction

Barbara seemed to have very typical hay fever but there were features that made it unlikely that hers was a straightforward case. The effect on her life, however, was serious. Considerable medical investigation was required before the problem was solved.

Personal details

Name Barbara Edelman. Unmarried
Age 33
Occupation Senior executive of a small public relations firm
Family one brother. Both parents alive and well

Medical background

Barbara has always enjoyed excellent health. She is an ambitious young woman who works hard and keeps herself fit by playing tennis in the summer and squash in the winter. She has had no serious illnesses and the only feature of her medical background was a fracture of her right tibia and fibula in a skiing accident when she was 22.

The present complaint

For no apparent reason Barbara has begun to have severe attacks of congestion of the nose, burning in her throat with a choking sensation. There is nasal catarrh with a frequent post-nasal drip. These attacks affect her voice and make it very difficult for her to interview clients comfortably. She is embarrassed by the constant necessity to clear her throat and annoyed at the loss of her usual voice resonance.

The history

The doctor is uncertain of the cause of these symptoms, which are not related to the seasons, but occur at regular intervals. He asks some more questions and Barbara tells him that the attacks are worst in the mornings, that they occur for a few days only every few weeks. She also admits that during the attacks she also has some slight irritation and watering of her eyes. The doctor then enquires into Barbara's personal and family history. Has she or any close relative ever had hay fever, eczema, asthma or nettle-rash? Barbara is a little surprised at these questions but assures him that there is no such history.

Next, he asks about domestic pets. Does Barbara have a cat or a dog? No. The doctor then asks Barbara how often she vacuum cleans her mattress. Barbara considers this rather impertinent but assures him that this is done regularly. The doctor explains that this question is related to the possibility that the problem could be due to house dust mites or their droppings.

The doctor examines Barbara's throat and then inspects the inside of her nose using a torch and a metal speculum to keep each nostril wide open in turn. He informs Barbara that everything appears to be entirely normal, and that the probability is that she is simply suffering from repeated colds. He prescribes some decongestant nose drop. Barbara is dubious but accepts this advice.

Two months later she is back again, insisting that her attacks are not common colds. The doctor decides to refer her to an allergist.

The management in hospital

In the out-patient department the specialist takes a detailed history and agrees with Barbara that she is not having colds. She tells her that her attacks are almost certainly caused by an allergy and takes a sample of blood for an IgE assessment. At her second visit Barbara is told by the specialist that her IgE levels are unusually high, even for a person with severe hay fever. She explains that IgE is the type of antibody associated with allergic reactions such as hay fever, asthma and urticaria. The problem now is to discover the particular allergen that is causing the attacks. She therefore marks a number of little circles on Barbara's arm with a pen and opposite each writes a word such as 'grass', 'tree', 'fungus', 'fur', 'dander' and so on. The specialist now brings out a range of small labelled bottles containing extracts of various substances. With the glass rods attached to the stoppers she puts a drop of each in the appropriate circle and then, quite gently, pricks through the drop into the skin with sharp needles. Barbara is then asked to sit in the waiting room for 15 minutes.

The doctor's comments

When Barbara returns with an unchanged arm, the allergist looks a little puzzled. She tells her that none of the common allergens are responsible and that a special test will have to be done. This is called a *radio-allergo-sorbent test*, or RAST for short. This test can actually determine the specific form of IgE that the patient is producing and thus identify the allergen. She takes a blood sample and asks Barbara to come back in two weeks' time. During this period Barbara has another severe attack.

On her next visit the allergist tells Barbara that she has solved the problem. 'Your allergy is due to a rather unexpected cause, a mite called *Lepidoglyphus destructor*. This has been found in farm barns, storage areas generally, building sites, bakeries and in damp houses.'

Barbara insists that she has been to no such places. The allergist tells her that it must be somewhere she goes to every few weeks as the attacks occur at such intervals. She also tells her that the mite lives on fungi but that these may not be apparent. Barbara insists that this could not possibly be the cause of her problems.

'Don't you go regularly to a bakery, or perhaps some sort of store?' asks the doctor.

'I get my bread from Sainsbury's . . .' Suddenly, Barbara stops. 'The attic!' she says. 'Could it possibly be the attic? It is a bit mouldy. And I do have to go up there every few weeks because I haven't room for . . .'

'I suspect we've found the answer,' said the allergist.

The follow-up

This was indeed the case. The allergist was interested enough in this unusual case to arrange for samples to be taken from the attic dust and *Lepidoglyphus destructor* was identified by an entomological colleague. Barbara had been thinking about having an attic conversion done and this finding tipped the balance. The place was cleared, a great deal of junk thrown away, the area vacuum cleaned, the wood treated and an architect and builder approached.

From the time the attic was cleared and converted Barbara has had no further attacks.

Other IgE tests

It is not often necessary actually to find out what kind of IgE is being produced in the body of a hay fever sufferer. But when this is the only way to be sure of the diagnosis, the doctor has a choice of methods by which the IgE can be identified. These are clever laboratory tests that were originally worked out to identify immunoglobulins (antibodies) for other purposes but which can equally well be used to investigate IgE. The essential point on which all these tests depend is that any particular antigen – and there are many thousands of these, all different – will result in the production by the body of only its own particular and identifiable protein immunoglobulin (antibody). This antibody will link on only to its own specific antigen. This being so, if you have a sample of the antigen – whether this is on a virus, bacterium, cell, worm parasite, pollen grain or whatever – you can check whether the body of the person concerned has previously been 'challenged' by the antigen. In other words, whether the person has had a particular infection or infestation or allergy.

All these special tests depend on checking, in various ways, whether a known antigen combines with its particular specific antibody. This can be done by labelling antigens with a radioactive element, or by linking them with a dye that will fluoresce under ultraviolet light, or in other ways.

The ELISA test

Nowadays, the most popular test of this kind is called the *ELISA test*. ELISA stands for *Enzyme-Linked ImmunoSorbent Assay*. This test is used for so many purposes that it is worth describing in some detail. It is, for instance, currently the standard test for HIV infection. People who are HIV positive will almost certainly have had an ELISA test.

The test detects the antibodies to the particular infection it is intended to look for and requires a known sample of the suspected organism or allergen (which bears the antigen). This sample is stuck onto a hollow in a plastic plate and any unstuck material is washed off. The blood serum is then added to the plate. If the antibody is present it will link firmly to the antigen. A solution is now added containing a substance called a *ligand* that can attach to any kind of antibody and that is chemically linked to a chemical activator (an enzyme) called *peroxidase*. The plate is again washed. The presence of the antibody now means that the enzyme is present. This enzyme, if present, will cause a colour change in a solution, called *chromogen*, which is now added. The enzyme is, of course, retained only if the specific antibody is present and has attached itself to the antigen stuck to the plate. When this is so the *enzyme* operates and the colour changes. This is the indication of a positive result.

The ELISA test can detect antibodies to almost anything. It is capable, for instance, of identifying allergens on all kinds of different pollens, on house and other mites of various species, on mite faeces, on animal skin scales or fur, on a wide range of fungal spores, and so on. Kits, for pathology laboratories, are produced to identify a very wide range of antibodies. To perform the ELISA test for the diagnosis of AIDS infection, it is necessary to have a sample of the AIDS virus, the human immunodeficiency virus, as the antigen; to perform the test for allergies, samples of the various possible allergens are needed.

Differential diagnosis

This impressive sounding phrase is used by doctors to indicate the process by which a selection is made from the list of possible conditions from which a patient might be suffering. Any given set of symptoms and signs might suggest more than one disease – sometimes several. Accurate diagnosis is essential if the best available treatment is to be provided. This is why doctors are always uneasy if they find themselves trying to treat a disease without knowing precisely what it is.

The differential diagnosis of hay fever is not particularly difficult as there are not many conditions that so closely resemble it as to cause much confusion. This is especially true of seasonal allergic rhinitis (see Chapter 1), but the range widens if the condition is non-seasonal.

Possible causes of confusion, in addition to the common cold, include:

- the condition *vasomotor rhinitis* that features frequent runny nose and nasal congestion for no very obvious reason. This is not an allergic disorder;
- *rhinitis medicamentosa*, a condition caused by various drugs such as aspirin, oral contraceptives, reserpine and hydralazine as well as the 'rebound' effect of drugs used locally as drops or sprays to *reduce* nasal congestion (decongestants);
- nasal congestion due to sudden changes of temperature or humidity;
- nasal congestion due to exposure to strong-smelling and irritant vapours;
- runny nose, watering eyes and sweating as a result of taking

unduly spicy or physically hot food. This is called *gustatory rhinitis*;
- nasal congestion from alcoholic overindulgence;
- nasal congestion from long-sustained sexual excitement, especially in men.

The last of these is included mainly for interest. It has been widely suggested, possibly on the basis of individual experience, that the nasal mucous membrane is an erectile tissue that may respond in this way to sexual arousal. There is no denying that it has an excellent blood supply, but it seems fanciful to equate it with the spongy erectile tissue of the penis or the clitoris.

5
Perennial Allergic Rhinitis

Perennial allergic rhinitis (PAR) is not really hay fever, but the symptoms are almost identical. The real difference between PAR and true hay fever is that the former can occur at any time of the year and commonly occurs all the year round. The latter is, of course, seasonal and occurs only when pollens and spores are carried in the atmosphere. In every other respect, including the symptoms (see Chapter 3) and the whole of the immunological process involved (see Chapter 2), the two conditions are the same. PAR can be just as severe as hay fever and, because it can occur at any time, is often more disabling.

The allergens

PAR has many more possible causes than hay fever. If you are prone to allergies, it is important that you should have an idea of the range of allergens that can cause it. The following list is far from complete, because no one knows all the substances that can cause PAR. New allergens are constantly being discovered. The list does, however, contain the commonest and most important of the known allergens:

- household dust mites;
- dust mite excreta;
- cockroach excreta;
- insect parts;
- organic fibres and lint;
- domestic animal skin flakes (dander);
- animal fur;
- fungal spores from mouldy hay;
- weevil-infested wheat flour;
- *Penicillium* spores from mouldy cheese;
- cat saliva;

- silverfish;
- dust lice;
- pyrethrum (used as an insecticide);
- orris root;
- flax seed;
- cotton seed;
- vegetable gums;
- pigeon droppings;
- budgerigar droppings;
- mushroom compost;
- cork dust;
- woodpulp;
- hairdressing chemicals such as ammonium persulphate;
- various drugs in powder form;
- industrial enzymes;
- bee, wasp and other insect stings.

All these allergens are proteins or carry proteins. It is always the proteins that cause the trouble. You will see that some of these allergens are likely to be encountered in the home environment while others are more likely to be picked up at work. In the case of the industrial allergens, the risk to casual visitors, such as customers in a hairdressing salon, is very small. People who work in environments in which PAR allergens are present are, however, in danger of developing an allergic rhinitis, especially if they already have atopy (see Chapter 2).

Domestic mites

The most important human allergens causing PAR are the household mites and their products. This has been proved by a great deal of research. Of the many species of mites, the most important are *Dermatophagoides farinae* and *Dermatophagoides pteronyssinus*. If you know a little Greek you will have worked out that this genus of mite lives by eating skin. *Derma-* is Greek for 'skin' and *phagos-* means 'eating' (as in *phagocyte*). So far as we know, flakes of human skin are the principal source of nourishment of these tiny creatures. So as to feed most comfortably, house mites live in bedding, mattresses, pillows, soft toys, upholstery and carpets. They appreciate a nice warm atmosphere and reproduce most actively at temperatures between 18°C and 21°C (65°F to 70°F). They also prefer a relative humidity of at least 50 per cent.

Dermatophagoides species are so small that they are barely visible to the naked eye and are seldom seen. They are about 0.5 millimetres 1/50 inches long. The allergen that causes the most trouble is not carried by the mite itself but occurs on its faeces. These are coated with a thick layer of the protein enzymes they use for digestion and it is one of these proteins that acts mainly as the allergen. Interestingly, the faecal protein allergen that causes most trouble is a digestive enzyme used by the mite to break down the skin protein it has eaten. If mites are present, the allergen is present.

The fact that the main allergen is on the mite faeces is important, because the balls of faeces are relatively heavy and do not readily float in the air as do pollen grains. They do, however, become airborne for half an hour or so if bedding is shaken or during household cleaning. The use of vacuum cleaners (through which these faecal balls can usually pass) also causes a brief airborne episode. These are the main ways in which this particular potent allergen gets into the noses of adults.

It has been found that children's soft toys are commonly heavily infested with *D. pteronyssinus*, so children with PAR may be getting the allergen directly from such toys. The number of mites on a given area of soft toy is likely to be two-and-a-half times as great as on a bed mattress. There is, however, one very effective and safe way of dealing with mites on soft toys such as teddy bears – put the toy in the freezer and leave it there for a few hours. Teddy bears don't have enough water in them to freeze solid and soon recover from the experience. The mites, however, don't.

Studies have shown that mites are more prevalent if a bedroom is occupied by more than one child and if the bedroom is damp. Other research has also shown that children with severe allergic problems are greatly improved if taken to Alpine regions at altitudes above 1,000 metres. At such altitudes, the air is so dry that mites cannot survive. It was, incidentally, the observation of this fact that first drew attention to the significance of house mites in PAR.

Other species of mite incriminated in causing PAR include the storage mites *Tyrophagus longior*, *Acarus farris* and *Lepidoglyphus destructor* and mites from the *Euroglyptus* and *Cheyletus* genera. Almost certainly many others are involved. Scientists recognize some 30,000 different species of mites, and this is probably about one-tenth of all those that exist, so there are plenty to choose from.

Domestic animals

The main cat allergens come from cat saliva and cat skin. Cats deposit large quantities of saliva on their fur in the course of washing. This saliva, which contains a small proportion of protein organic matter, quickly dries and the organic content is released into the domestic atmosphere. Because of this, and because most cats wash frequently, the air of cat loving households is fairly constantly loaded with cat saliva allergens. These protein allergens are very small and light, and remain for long periods in the air. They are an important cause of PAR. Cat skin scales (dander) and hair particles also become readily airborne.

It has been shown that levels of these allergens can be substantially reduced if the human owners accept the responsibility for cat washing. It is unnecessary to use the same methods as the cat; a weekly wash with a mild baby shampoo, although unpopular with the cat, can solve the PAR problem for some people. Many owners, allergic to animal fur, dander or saliva, will have a fairly shrewd suspicion of the cause but may be reluctant to admit it for fear of being advised to dispose of their pets.

Dog hair does not appear to be a significant allergen. Saliva, dander and dried urine, however, are common causes of PAR. Again, regular washing is recommended.

Other insect allergens

Domestically, the most important of these seem to be cockroach products and parts. Cockroaches are highly successful colonizers of urban environments and are present in most buildings, both in the tropics and in temperate regions. They are especially prevalent where sources of food are available to them and are adept at concealing themselves. Hundreds of cockroaches can hide in a kitchen that appears to be wholly uninhabited. They prefer a warm, humid and dark habitat and live off almost anything organic, especially food scraps, paper, books, clothing and dead insects. Females commonly deposit 50 batches of 16 eggs during a lifetime of 18 months and these hatch after 45 days.

Cockroach excreta and the powdered debris from dead cockroaches and their insect prey can readily become airborne to act as nasal allergens and cause PAR. If you live exclusively in an urban area and suffer from unexplained perennial allergic rhinitis, you should certainly consider the possibility that your problem is due to this cause. The cockroaches may be present in your home or, perhaps more likely, in your place of work.

Very determined efforts are needed to deal with cockroach infestations and it is unlikely that you will succeed in eradicating the nuisance without professional help. Studies have shown that only spraying by properly trained and well informed pest control specialists is likely to be successful.

Treatment

The most important element in the treatment of PAR involves the removal of the allergen, or, if that is not possible, separation of the sufferer from it. Treatment of the symptoms is also important. Symptomatic treatment is identical to the treatment of seasonal allergic rhinitis (hay fever) and you can read all about that in Chapters 9 and 10.

6
All About Antihistamines

It is probably true to say that antihistamine drugs are the mainstay of the management of hay fever and PAR. Antihistamines are certainly used more widely than any other class of drugs to treat hay fever. And now that many of them are available to you over-the-counter without prescription, there is much you can do for yourself to alleviate your hay fever symptoms.

There is a convention in naming drugs that the 'official' or *generic* name is spelled with a lower case initial. Trade names, on the other hand, are capitalized. This convention is followed in this book. For every generic name there are usually several, sometimes scores, of trade names for the same stuff. It is worth checking the generic names of your favourite medications so that if one preparation is unavailable you may possibly be able to obtain an identical substitute under another name.

You already know quite a lot about histamine, but to understand fully how the antihistamine drugs work it is necessary to review the actions of this unpleasant substance and to learn more about how it causes so much trouble to so many people.

More about the effects of histamine

We have seen that histamine has several actions:

- to widen small blood vessels;
- to cause the smallest vessels to leak fluid;
- as a result to lead to waterlogging (oedema) of tissues;
- to narrow air tubes;
- to stimulate sensory nerves so as to cause strong discomfort, irritation and itching;
- to cause glands to secrete.

Histamine has two other effects that have not yet been mentioned. It is a powerful stimulant of stomach acid and it is used by the brain and nervous system to carry messages. The action of histamine on the brain is not fully understood but we do know quite a lot about it. We know that too much histamine causes a severe headache and that smaller quantities are necessary in the brain for normal brain function and the maintenance of full consciousness. The latter effect is best shown by what happens when histamine is prevented from acting in the brain by the action of antihistamines.

The molecules of histamine operate by locking into certain action sites, on the surface of cells, called histamine receptors. These are present on cells all over the body and are of three types. Those we are concerned with here are found especially on cells such as the smooth muscle cells of arteries and air tubes, the cells of the nose lining generally, and on the brain cells.

How antihistamines work

Antihistamine drugs were first discovered as early as 1937. Unfortunately, the first known antihistamine turned out to be much too poisonous to be used as a medicine. By 1944, however, the much safer drug *pyrilamine maleate* had been developed. By the early 1950s many useful and safe antihistamines had been developed. These drugs are chemically similar to histamine in that they fit neatly into the receptor sites, but they differ from histamine in that, although occupying the sites, they do not act on the cells in the way that histamine does. In fact, they do not act on the cells at all. They are just like plugs; they fill the sites but don't activate the cells. The whole point of this is, of course, that if the histamine receptor sites are all already occupied by the antihistamine drug molecules, it really doesn't matter how much histamine is swilling about in the area – it simply cannot get to the receptors to have its usual effects.

Until recently it was believed, and with good reason, that this was all that the antihistamines did. Indeed, until a range of new antihistamines (the 'second generation' antihistamines) was developed, this probably was all that they did. Some of the new drugs, however, while acting very efficiently as receptor site blockers, do seem to have another very useful effect. Drugs such as *terfenadine* actually manage to limit the release of histamine from mast cells. All in all, antihistamines are highly effective in controlling the symptoms of hay fever and PAR.

Antihistamines and the brain

Antihistamines that get to the brain, to block the histamine receptor sites there, prevent the normal neurotransmitter action of histamine. This has a good effect and a not-so-good effect. The good news is that blocking histamine action on the brain can cure, or at least greatly alleviate motion sickness. The snag is that the person concerned can become quite sleepy. Sleepiness is probably the principal undesired side-effect of antihistamine drugs. Only certain antihistamines are used in this way; others are not recommended for children. Some antihistamines are so effective in blocking nerve transmission that they can even be used as local anaesthetics.

Because there has been a great demand for antihistamines that did *not* cause sleepiness, research scientists decided to look rather closely at the reason why some drugs seemed to be able to get from the bloodstream into the brain while others did not. Drugs in the blood get to the cells of the body by passing through the walls of the smallest blood vessels – the single-cell-layered capillaries. Studies of the blood capillaries in the brain showed that they were different from capillaries elsewhere. While capillaries in the body generally had quite large pores between their cells, those in the brain had cells fused tightly together. If a drug molecule was large, it could get through the walls of the body capillaries with no trouble but it might be prevented from getting through the walls of the capillaries in the brain.

If you look at the chemical formulae of the second generation antihistamine drugs you will see that most of them have larger and more complex molecules than those of the earlier antihistamines. Most experts believe that the absence of sedating and other nervous system effects of some of these newer antihistamines, especially terfenadine, is due to the fact that they are unable to get through the walls of the brain capillaries, or, as doctors express it, cannot pass through the 'blood–brain barrier'.

Length of action of antihistamines

Antihistamine drugs are well absorbed when taken by mouth and are not broken down by stomach acid. The peak levels in the blood occur two to three hours after they are taken. The useful effects on symptoms, however, start within an hour and the greatest effects start five to seven hours after taking the dose.

Antihistamines act for much longer than the time they are present in the blood. For example, after a one-week course of some of them, an appreciable effect persists for another seven days. In an emergency, antihistamines can be given by injection directly into the bloodstream. This produces an almost immediate effect. Some of the more recent antihistamines dissolve poorly in water, however, and are not available in injectable form, so the earlier, more soluble drugs are used.

There is no evidence that long-term use of antihistamines in any way reduces their effectiveness or the rate at which they are eliminated from the body. Tolerance to the sedative effects of some antihistamines may, however, develop, so this can become less of a problem with time. Unfortunately, you can't rely on this happening with all of them.

One thing you should note – exceeding the recommended dosage does not increase the effect. Careful trials have shown that even doubling the standard dosage does not produce a significant increase in the relief of symptoms. An increase in dosage could be dangerous, however, so don't try it.

Side-effects of antihistamines

It is important that you should be aware of the possible effects of antihistamines. The commonest and most troublesome of these is sedation. This shows itself by sleepiness, general slowing and lengthened reaction time. Note that this can be greatly worsened by alcohol and that the combination can be dangerous. You might, for instance, find yourself prosecuted for 'driving under the influence' after taking only one or two drinks if you are also taking antihistamines. The law will not excuse you on the grounds that the medication is justified. Some antihistamines are so strongly sedative that they are used for this purpose, especially in children. These selected antihistamines are considered the safest sedatives for children.

Some of the more recent second generation antihistamines do not reach the brain as easily as others and so have little or no sedative effect. The antihistamines that are available over-the-counter are said to be non-sedating, but you should be careful all the same.

Other possible side effects of antihistamines that you should be aware of include:

- diminished alertness;
- slowing of mental activity;
- blurring of vision;
- dry mouth;
- difficulty with urination;
- digestive upsets;
- constipation;
- headache;
- impotence;
- disorientation;
- sometimes paradoxical stimulation;
- dizziness;
- weight gain;
- heart irregularities;
- skin rashes.

Apart from the effects on alertness, none of these side effects are particularly common. Note that side-effects may occur with one person but not with another. If they occur in your case you should simply avoid that particular drug. There is no question of treating side-effects.

There are a few other points to note in this context. You should be rather careful with antihistamines if you suffer from angle-closure (narrow-angle) glaucoma or if you have an enlarged prostate gland so that it takes you longer to empty your bladder than it used to. If you are an epileptic or have any form of liver disease you should also be careful. If you do have any of these conditions it would be as well to discuss the matter with your doctor before deciding to treat yourself with antihistamines.

In general, antihistamines are remarkably safe. *Large* overdosage with antihistamines can, however, be very dangerous and can lead to:

- involuntary jerky movements (*dyskinesia*);
- severe muscle spasm (*dystonia*);
- heart irregularities;
- heart block;
- epileptic-type seizures;
- hallucinations;
- psychotic episodes;
- coma;
- death.

Clearly, this is not to be risked. So antihistamines, like other drugs, should be kept out of reach of depressed people and children. Overdosage is treated by inducing vomiting and giving activated charcoal. This helps to reduce the absorption of the drug.

A report published in June 1994 indicated that at that time it was not yet known which of the antihistamines was safest for use during pregnancy. As a general rule, all drugs are to be avoided during the early weeks of pregnancy when the major structures and organs of the fetus are being formed.

Some representative antihistamine drugs

Trade names are capitalized. You can find the generic name of the drug you are using on the packaging.

acrivastine A second generation antihistamine. Used to treat hay fever and nettle rash (*urticaria*). It is taken by mouth. Possible side-effects include drowsiness, but this is rare. A trade name is *Semprex*.

antazoline Used to treat allergic conjunctivitis. It is taken in the form of eye drops. It also has weak local anaesthetic effects. A trade name is *Antistin-Privine*.

astemizole A second generation antihistamine. Used to treat hay fever and allergic skin conditions. It is taken by mouth. Possible side-effects include weight gain and, on very high dosage, heart irregularity. A trade name is *Hismanal*.

Atarax A trade name for *hydroxyzine hydrochloride*.

azatadine A second generation antihistamine. Used to treat hay fever, urticaria, itching and stings. It is taken by mouth. Possible side-effects include drowsiness, slowed reaction time, headache, nausea and either increase of, or loss of, appetite. A trade name is *Optimine*.

azelastine Taken as a metered dose nasal spray for the treatment of hay fever. Possible side-effects include nasal irritation and disturbances of taste sensation. A trade name is *Rhinolast*.

brompheniramine Used to treat hay fever and perennial allergic rhinitis. It is taken by mouth as tablets or a liquid. A trade name is *Dimotane Plus*.

chlorpheniramine Used to treat hay fever, perennial allergic rhinitis and anaphylactic shock. It is taken by mouth or by injection. Trade names are *Aller-chlor*, *Haymine*, *Piriton*, *Phenetron*.

Clarityn A trade name for *loratadine*.

clemastine Used to treat hay fever and perennial allergic rhinitis. It is taken by mouth as tablets or a liquid. A trade name is *Tavegil*.

cyproheptadine Used to treat allergic disorders generally including itchy skin conditions. It is taken by mouth. Possible side-effects include stimulation of appetite, interactions with monoamine oxidase inhibitors (see Chapter 7 – decongestants), drowsiness, etc. A trade name is *Periactin*.

Daneral A trade name for *pheniramine*.

dimethindine maleate Used to treat hay fever, urticaria and other allergic conditions. It is taken by mouth. Possible side-effects include drowsiness and slowed reactions. A trade name is *Vibrocil*.

Dimotane Plus A trade name for *brompheniramine*.

Haymine A trade name for *chlorpheniramine*.

Hismanal A trade name for *astemizole*.

hydroxyzine hydrochloride Used mainly to relieve itching in nettle rash and other skin conditions. It is taken my mouth. A trade name is *Atarax*.

ketotifen A second generation antihistamine. Used to treat allergic rhinitis and allergic conjunctivitis. This drug can stabilize mast cells and reduce histamine release. Possible side-effects include drowsiness, dizziness, dry mouth and, occasionally, jumpiness. A trade name is *Zaditen*.

loratadine A second generation antihistamine. Used to treat hay fever and perennial allergic rhinitis. It is taken by mouth. Possible side-effects include headache, fatigue and nausea. A trade name is *Clarityn*.

mequitazine Used to treat hay fever and perennial allergic rhinitis. It is taken by mouth. A trade name is *Primalan*.

Optimine A trade name for *azatadine*.

oxatomide Used to treat hay fever. It is taken by mouth. A trade name is *Tinset*.

Periactin A trade name for *cyproheptadine*.

Phenergan A trade name for *promethazine*.

phenindamine Used to treat allergic conditions. It is taken by mouth. A trade name is *Thephorin*.

pheniramine Used to control allergic reactions generally. It is taken by mouth. A trade name is *Daneral*.

Piriton A trade name for *chlorpheniramine*.

Primalan A trade name for *mequitazine*.

Pro-Actidil A trade name for *triprolidine*.

promethazine Used for allergies, nausea and vomiting, travel sickness and as a sedative in children. It is taken by mouth as tablet or a liquid. A trade name is *Phenergan*.

Rhinocort A trade name for *budesonide*.

Rhinolast A trade name for *azelastine*.

Semprex A trade name for *acrivastine*.

Sinutab Antihistamine A trade name for a compound of the pain killer *paracetamol*, the decongestant *pseudoephedrine* and *chlorpheniramine*.

Tavegil A trade name for *clemastine*.

terfenadine A second generation antihistamine. Used to treat allergic rhinitis and urticaria. It is taken by mouth. Possible side-effects include digestive upset, skin rashes, sweating, heart irregularity. A trade name is *Triludan*.

Thephorin A trade name for *phenindamine*.

Tinset A trade name for *oxatomide*.

Triludan A trade name for *terfenadine*.

trimeprazine Used to relieve itching in allergic conditions and as a sedative for children. A trade name is *Vallergan*.

triprolidine Used to treat allergy and to relieve the symptoms of colds. It is taken by mouth. Possible side-effects include drowsiness, slowed reaction time and, rarely, skin rashes. Trade names are *Actidil*, *Actifed* and *Pro-Actidil*.

Ucerax A trade name for *hydroxyzine hydrochloride*.

Vallergan A trade name for *trimeprazine*.

Zatiden A trade name for *ketotifen*.

7
Other Forms of Treatment

Anthihistamines are by no means the only way of dealing with hay fever and PAR. Some of the other forms of treatment are even more effective than the antihistamines. Unfortunately, the more active a drug or procedure, the more likely it is to have side-effects or other disadvantages, so you have to balance one thing against another. Here are the essential points about the other ways of managing these conditions.

Steroids

Steroids, or, more correctly, *glucocorticoids*, are natural body substances without which we would be in real trouble. They are essential for the normal and safe running of the body, and the amounts produced – by the adrenal glands on top of the kidneys – vary considerably depending on the body's needs.

Many people feel very unhappy at the idea of taking steroids. This is because they have heard alarming tales of the terrible things that steroids, used as drugs, can cause:

- stunting of the growth of children;
- osteoporosis;
- spontaneous fractures;
- breakdown of healed ulcers;
- a shut-down of the body's own steroid production;
- interference with the immune system so that latent infections are reactivated and new infections such as thrush encouraged.

All these things *can* happen and, in people who are receiving large doses of steroids by mouth or injection over long periods of time, sometimes do happen. Treatment of this kind is called *systemic* treatment because high levels of the drugs pass to almost all parts of the body. But in the management of hay fever and

PAR there is no question of systemic treatment. If steroids are used, they are used locally (*topically*), nearly always in the form of nasal sprays.

In fact, steroids are the most powerful and effective drugs available for the treatment and control of hay fever and PAR. Used topically, they are every bit as effective as if taken by mouth or injection and are far safer. For years doctors have considered steroids as a kind of fall-back or last resort to be used when everything else fails, but this view is now beginning to change.

One reason for this is the discovery that steroids, used at the beginning of the hay fever season actually prevent the accumulation of mast cells in the nose lining. If you have read Chapter 2 carefully, there will be no need to emphasize how important this is. No mast cells – no hay fever or PAR. Steroids cannot, of course, be relied on to eliminate mast cells completely but, properly used, their effect can be remarkable.

Secondly, steroids are the most powerful anti-inflammatory drugs available and can be relied on to cut down, or even eliminate, the inflammation caused by histamine and other mast cell granule products. Thirdly, steroids interfere with the unfortunate progressive increase in sensitivity to allergens that so often results in hay fever and PAR getting steadily worse.

The steroids most commonly used are *Syntaris* (*flunisolide*), *Aerobec, Beconase* or *Beclazone* (*beclomethasone*) and *Dexarhinaspray* (*dexamethasone*). It is important to use these in exactly the prescribed dosage. A usual instruction might be two sprays (50µg) of flunisolide in each nostril twice a day or one spray (42µg) of beclomethasone in each nostril two to four times a day. You should try to use as little as is necessary to keep the problem under control. It is only fair to say that it is possible to detect slight general effects with normal dosage of dexamethasone nasal sprays. The experts report that no general side-effects have been detected with nasal use of flunisolide and beclomethasone.

These steroids can, however, have certain side-effects within the nose itself. The main problem is a feeling of irritation and burning for a while after using the spray. In some people, perhaps one in fifty, the irritation is severe enough to promote a nosebleed. A very occasional user will even develop a hole in the thin partition between the two sides of the nose (*perforated nasal septum*). This is not particularly serious and will usually eventually heal. Very occasionally a patient might develop a thrush infection of the inside of the nose. This is rare and can be effectively treated.

Decongestants

Congestion (stuffiness) of the nose is an unpleasant feature of hay fever and PAR. It is often so extreme that the nasal air passages are completely closed and you have to resort to mouth breathing. This is not particularly good for health as you are then taking unconditioned air into your lungs. Decongestant drugs are those that act on blood vessels, causing the tiny muscles in their walls to tighten so that they are narrowed and less blood can flow through them. As a result, the vein sinuses under the mucous membrane lining collapse and the lining flattens. If this is not quite clear, read the section on the nose in Chapter 2.

Nasal decongestant drugs are called *alpha-adrenergic blockers*. This name simply means that they prevent an adrenaline-like hormone from acting at certain receptor sites on the muscles in the blood vessel and elsewhere. They have a double effect. As well as shrinking the nose lining they can counteract the sleepiness caused by antihistamines. They work most quickly and effectively when used directly on the nose lining as drops or a spray, such as *Medihaler*, but this method has two great disadvantages. With repeated use, the duration of the effect becomes less; and when the effect wears off there is a strong tendency for the congestion to get at least as bad as it was before, if not worse. This is called *rebound congestion*.

For these reasons decongestants are, on the whole, best taken by mouth in carefully limited dosage. The nasal spray preparation can, however, be useful to let you get off to sleep and to open up the nasal passages briefly so as to let the aerosol from a steroid spray get to the parts it would not otherwise reach. Doctors also use them to permit proper examination of the nose.

If you use decongestants by mouth – usually *pseudoephedrine* or *phenylpropanolamine* in the form of tablets, capsules or mixtures – you may experience certain effects resulting from the action of the drug on other adrenaline receptors in your body. Adrenaline-like or amphetamine-like effects such as jumpiness, irritability, overactivity and insomnia are quite familiar to people taking oral decongestants. You may find these unpleasant.

It is also important for you to appreciate that these effects can actually be dangerous if you have heart disease or high blood pressure or if you are epileptic or have an overactive thyroid gland. They are especially risky if you are being treated for depression or other conditions with a drug of the monoamine oxidase (MAO) inhibitor group. If you are on such a drug your doctor will have warned you to avoid cheese, wine, chocolate, yeasts and other foods. Commonly prescribed monoamine oxidase inhibitor drugs include *Nardil* (*phenelzine*), *Marplan* (*isocarboxazid*), *Parnate* or *Parstelin* (*tranylcypromine*) and *Manerix* (*moclobemide*). While taking these MAO inhibitor drugs, oral decongestants can cause your blood pressure to rise to a dangerous level.

In view of these facts it is best to take medical advice before using oral decongestant drugs.

Cromoglycate

The drug *cromoglycate*, also known as *cromolyn sodium*, has a very useful effect in preventing degranulation of mast cells (see Chapter 2). The way it does this is still uncertain. Most accounts refer to 'stabilization of the mast cell membrane' but this idea is no longer so confidently held. From your point of view what matters is that it works. The drug, prescribed most commonly under the trade name of *Intal*, is widely used in inhalers for the control of asthma. Intal is available as a nasal spray and should be used from the beginning of the allergy season, preferably before any symptoms occur.

Some people get an excellent result from cromoglycate; others do not. The drug is very safe and there are hardly any side-effects. The main disadvantage is that it has to be used four to six times a day. Intal is not a steroid or an antihistamine and is certainly worth trying. Note, however, that some preparations, such as *Intal Compound*, also contain an adrenaline-like decongestant. Remember that cromoglycate cannot, and will not, deal with symptoms due to histamine already released from mast cell granules. Its only mode of action is to prevent these unpleasant substances from being released.

If you are greatly troubled by watering and redness of the eyes from hay fever, you can use cromoglycate in the form of eye drops such as *Opticrom* or *Eye-Crom*.

Some representative non-antihistamine drugs

beclomethasone Steroid drug. Used to treat hay fever and PAR. It is taken as a nasal spray. A trade name is *Beconase*.

Beconase A trade name for beclomethasone.

budesonide Steroid drug. Used to treat hay fever and PAR. It is taken by nasal spray. A trade name is *Rhinocort*.

cromoglycate An anti-inflammatory drug that prevents the release of histamine from mast cells. It is taken as a nasal spray or drops. A trade name is *Nalcrom*.

Flixonase A trade name for the corticosteroid drug *fluticasone propionate* used as a metered dose spray inhaler to prevent and treat hay fever. May cause irritation to the nose, nosebleeds or may cause upsets of taste and smell.

flunisolide A steroid drug. Used to treat hay fever and PAR. It is taken as a nasal spray. A trade name is *Syntaris*.

Intal A trade name for *sodium chromoglycate*.

Nalcrom A trade name for *cromoglycate*.

pseudoephedrine A powerful decongestant drug. Used to relieve nasal blockage and to facilitate access for other hay fever medication. See precautions mentioned in this chapter. Trade names are *Sudafed*, *Sudafed SA* and *Galpseud*.

Sudafed Plus A trade name for *triprolidine* and the decongestant drug *pseudoephedrine*.

Syntaris A trade name for the steroid *flunisolide*.

Triominic A mixture of the nasal decongestant drug *phenylpropanolamine* and the antihistamine drug *pheniramine*.

Desensitization

Desensitization is a method of treatment designed to boost the effectiveness of the immune system in combating hay fever and PAR. It is done by giving a series of injections of the very allergens that cause these disorders. Since these conditions are caused, in the first place, by a defect in the functioning of the immune system, you can see that any explanation of how desensitization works is likely to be complicated. The fact is that, to date, no one has been able to explain convincingly how it works. Even the latest textbooks of immunology have to admit that the process is not fully understood. We do know, however, that, in cases where it is effective, the levels of IgE eventually drop and those of the commoner antibody type IgG (gamma globulin) rise. IgG is said to be a *blocking antibody* that competes for the allergen, latches on to it and forms a complex that can be removed by phagocytes. IgG, of course, does not trigger degranulation of mast cells.

The first requirement is that there should be a precise diagnosis of the cause of the allergy so that the correct allergen can be given. This must then be made up in a very dilute solution suitable for injection. Injections of gradually increasing amounts of the allergen are given once or twice a week, just under the skin, until the doctor has reached the largest dose short of causing a general reaction. Injections of a substance to which you are known to be allergic can be very dangerous. For this reason, the process is to be undertaken only by someone who really knows what he or she is doing – in other words, a fully qualified scientific allergist. This is no job for self-styled 'allergists' or practitioners of alternative therapies.

It takes a long time for the desired effect to be achieved and you should not expect any benefit for at least three months. The injections are usually continued for two or three years. If all goes well, you should begin to become less allergic after the first three or four months and the improvement may then continue to increase progressively for up to two years. For these reasons, the course of injections is best started after the end of the hay fever season and then continued all the year round. They are given very carefully under close medical supervision to avoid severe reactions. If reactions occur they may be immediate or they may be delayed for four to six hours.

The danger of injecting allergens into allergic patients is neither slight nor fanciful. There was an average of one death per year in the UK from this cause over the period from 1959 to 1986. Most of these occurred in people being treated by non-specialists. When these facts became widely known, official disapproval of desensitization was expressed and the practice was largely abandoned. It is only recently that the real experts have again, in the light of increased knowledge, begun to consider the merits of this method of treatment.

A scheme of management

It will be useful to bring all this information together in a brief general account of the best way to manage your hay fever.

The first step is to be sure that you actually have hay fever or PAR. This means making an accurate diagnosis. Check Chapters 3 and 4 which cover symptoms and diagnosis. Next you should try to find out exactly what the allergen is that is causing your trouble. You may be able to do this for yourself simply by observing which particular grasses, tree pollens or fungal spores bring on your allergy. It will not be so easy to identify domestic allergens, but you can make some useful assumptions on the basis of frequency. Check Chapter 5 for details. If you are stuck on this one and simply have no idea of what is causing the allergy, you will have to try to persuade your doctor to arrange a skin prick test (see Chapter 4).

Once the background facts are established, you should do everything you can to avoid the allergen. See Chapter 11. If avoidance fails you are going to have to consider treatment. The first choice is between cromoglycate and an antihistamine. You should certainly use cromoglycate in the form of eye drops if you have much eye irritation with redness and watering. Cromoglycate by nasal spray, such as Rhynacrom, is also a good start but you will have to use it at least four times a day and it is rather expensive. No prescription is necessary.

It is difficult to advise on the choice of antihistamines because there are so many and because you can't really tell which will suit you best until you have tried. It is best to stick to the range recommended for hay fever or PAR rather than those used mainly for other purposes. Many of them are available without prescription.

If nasal congestion is a major feature you will probably need a decongestant. But do remember the possible dangers. Before considering decongestants, read the section above on these drugs. Use decongestants sparingly.

As to the use of steroid nasal sprays, you will have to make up your own mind. They are certainly effective and millions of people have used preparations such as Beconase with great satisfaction and with no indication of dangerous side-effects. You can get Beconase over-the-counter without prescription. Use two sprays in each nostril twice a day. You may find it worth while to read the section on steroids once again.

While on the subject of over-the-counter drugs, you should remember that a great many of these were, until fairly recently, available only on prescription. The fact that you can now buy them directly does not mean that they can safely be used casually or in doses greater than those recommended. To do so could be dangerous. If you need advice on any particular drug you are purchasing, you will usually find that the pharmacist will be glad to answer any of your questions. Pharmaceutical chemists are highly qualified and very well-informed people and often know at least as much about the actions and dangers of drugs as doctors.

The question of possible densensitization, and the management of any persistent complications (see Chapter 10), are matters for your doctor. Complications such as sinusitis or middle ear infection may require antibiotic treatment in addition to routine hay fever treatment. Antibiotics have no place in the management of uncomplicated hay fever or PAR.

8
The Emotional Dimension

Hay fever and perennial allergic rhinitis are not serious illnesses in the sense that cancer of the lung or coronary artery disease are serious. No one has ever died of hay fever. Nevertheless, these conditions are responsible for an enormous amount of distress to millions. This distress arises from interference with many aspects of life, especially human relationships.

It is difficult for those who have never experienced the embarrassments and discomforts of hay fever to understand why sufferers sometimes seem to make such a fuss about what is generally considered to be a minor disorder. Such people may be inclined to respond impatiently to a sufferer's refusal to visit a park or to go for a country walk. But there is nothing minor about a condition that makes it impossible to relate normally to other people.

Social activity

Young people in particular are affected by the emotional dimension in hay fever. Adolescents and young adults, already hypersensitive about their appearance, socially uncertain and easily embarrassed, are liable to become so self-conscious as a result of hay fever that they may prefer to give up social activity altogether rather than risk the humiliation of being seen by those they care about, sporting running red noses and red watery eyes, sneezing at frequent intervals and constantly fumbling with a handkerchief that is quickly becoming soaked. It is easy for others to smile at the social sensitivity of young people; to the sufferer it is all degrading, mortifying and deadly serious.

The purely subjective symptoms of hay fever – those that are not apparent to others such as the persistent soreness of the nose, the itching, pricking and burning in and around the nose and eyes, even severe pain in the face from the sinuses, also make effective socializing very difficult. It is not easy to be bright, lively, amusing or charming when you are feeling rotten, when your nose is blocked and your voice sounds ridiculously nasal to you.

Almost half of the women who suffer significantly from hay fever make the effort to carry on a normal social life. Men, always more sensitive in such matters, tend to opt out more readily. Only a fifth of men try to carry on with normal social relations. When both men and women sufferers are questioned, a fifth of them agree that their relations with others are affected at least to some extent. The sex life is particularly likely to be affected. Many avoid sex when affected. One person in fifty is driven by embarrassment, fastidiousness or even incapacity to a state of total chastity throughout the whole of the pollen season.

Hay fever and work

The same factors that disrupt social and sexual activity can operate to an even more marked extent in relation to work. In a social context you can, at least, excuse yourself and go home. This is more difficult if you are anxious to make the best possible impression on your boss and workmates. Hay fever can also so reduce your mental efficiency that you make silly and embarrassing mistakes. You are likely to believe, and you may well be right, that others are not going to make excuses for you on such trivial grounds as hay fever.

Sometimes the allergen is actually associated with the workplace so that the problems are made worse by going to work. If your job is connected with plants, grass, trees or other sources of allergen, your emotional reaction to your hay fever is likely to be severely exacerbated. If you are an adolescent sufferer and at a stage in your education when exams are of critical importance, you have every justification in feeling hard done by. Unfortunately, annual exams often coincide with the hay fever season. While your luckier colleagues are enjoying the benefits of the cool breezes wafting in from the school or college playing fields through the open windows, you may be sitting there just waiting for what you know will be a really horrible attack that may make it almost impossible for you to carry on writing that all-important paper.

Allergy and sex

The more severe forms of reaction to allergens, in particular asthma (Chapter 9) commonly have a serious effect on the sex life. Hay fever and PAR are less likely to cause major disruption of sexual activity, but they can certainly do so. Severe hay fever, of course, is a real blight on libido and it would be a determined partner who would insist. Aesthetic considerations apart, simple allergic rhinitis is, in itself, no bar to sex. PAR can, however, sometimes cause real problems. Here is a case history that illustrates the point.

Introduction

Walter is an orchestral cellist. He is a shy, lonely man who has never been successful with women. At last, however, he thinks he has found his ideal. Unfortunately, there is an unexpected problem.

Personal details

Name Walter Ainsworth
Age 44
Occupation Professional musician
Family Parents dead. No siblings

Medical background

Walter's general health has been reasonable, with no serious illnesses. He recollects being told that he suffered from eczema as a child, but he now has no skin problems. He finds it difficult to get as much exercise as he should and he is somewhat out of condition. He has always disliked seeing doctors, but his present problem has driven him to it.

The complaint

Walter visits his doctor with a complaint of sudden episodes of sore throat, coughing, sneezing, watering eyes, tightness in the chest and some wheeziness. He finds it particularly difficult to explain this complaint fully to his doctor and at first omits to mention an essential point – that the trouble arises only when he is making love to his fiancée. Fortunately, the doctor's questions are as persistent as they are pertinent and at last the whole story comes out. Walter has been dating Elizabeth for almost two years. Seven months ago they decided to get married. Walter has had no previous sexual experience but for some weeks now Elizabeth has been inviting him to spend the night with her in her flat.

At first, all went well and they had wonderful sex. But on the third or fourth occasion that he stayed overnight with her, he had one of these attacks and this has happened on every occasion since. He has become convinced that this is some kind of psychosomatic response to unconscious guilt. Elizabeth, too, is beginning to wonder whether something is wrong with their relationship. He and Elizabeth are, in fact, very much in love and ideally suited to one another. They are both very unhappy over this strange development.

The doctor asks whether Walter has ever had similar attacks anywhere other than in Elizabeth's flat. Walter assures him that he has not. The doctor then asks where exactly in the flat they make love. Walter shyly tells him that they always go to bed.

'Nowhere else,' says Walter.

'Have a go in the lounge,' advises the doctor, 'and report back to me.'

A week later Walter returns. He responds to the doctor's raised eyebrows with a gratified smile.

'All well?' asks the doctor.

'Wonderful,' says Walter. 'But I'm at a complete loss to understand why the place should make such a difference. Could it be a Freudian thing about bed?'

'Nonsense,' says the doctor, and explains that Walter is

suffering from a simple allergy to something present in the bedroom. He has a fairly shrewd idea what it is.

The investigation and diagnosis

The doctor then arranges for Walter to have skin prick sensitivity tests and diplomatically suggests that Walter bring Elizabeth with him when he returns for the results. Two weeks later the couple are in attendance.

The doctor explains that the tests have shown that Walter has developed an allergy to house mite faecal protein. It seems, he tells them, that the mites are in the bedding.

Elizabeth is horrified and embarrassed.

The doctor waves this aside and explains that nearly every house has mites. The remarkable thing is that Walter has, until now, escaped the allergy. Walter says he has always slept in nylon sheets. Could this be relevant?

'Certainly,' says the doctor, 'problem solved.'

The treatment

Elizabeth wants to burn all her bedding but the doctor laughs her out of this and advises her about high-temperature washes, miticides and, if necessary, plastic bags. Walter is given a prescription for Beconase and cromoglycate sprays. The doctor has become interested in the case and asks them to keep him posted as to progress.

The follow-up

Walter never has another attack. A month later the doctor receives an eloquent report in the form of a wedding invitation.

9
Hay Fever in Children

Hay fever is not common in very young children. This is because it normally takes years for a sufficient level of IgE to build up (see Chapter 2). Even so, the condition has been described in children as young as one year, and the number of cases rises steadily with increasing age. Children who develop hay fever are nearly always suffering from atopy (see Chapter 2) and commonly also have eczema. They are also prone to develop allergic asthma.

PAR commonly starts before the second year of life and is often associated with asthma. In such cases the allergen is usually the same for both conditions. Long-standing blockage of the nose in such children can lead to disturbances of the growth of the dental arches and irregularities in the way the teeth come together (*malocclusion*). Children suffer more from nasal blockage than adults because their nasal passages are relatively more narrow and can be obstructed by a lesser degree of swelling of the lining than in the case of adults.

Hay fever usually starts after the age of two and tends to become worse with each succeeding pollen season. In children, the most obvious signs are:

- mouth breathing;
- feeding difficulty because of blocked nose;
- snoring during sleep;
- a nasal tone to the voice;
- constant sniffing;
- nose picking;
- nosebleeds;
- nose rubbing;
- frequent sneezing;
- eye watering;
- redness of the eyes and eyelids;

- swelling around the eyes;
- a purplish discoloration around the eyes;
- a crease across the lower part of the nose (the 'allergic salute');
- undue tiredness;

Indications such as these should never be simply written off as 'a cold'. It is important to establish the diagnosis and to ensure that the child has proper treatment. Decongestive drops of pseudo-ephedrine or ephedrine can be very useful, but should not be used for more than a few days (see Chapter 7). Severe cases will probably need Beconase or cromoglycate nasal sprays.

Hay fever and PAR in children can sometimes have serious consequences.

The effect on the ears

Children affected in this way are more prone than average to the common childhood disorder of middle ear infection (*otitis media*). This is because of the ease with which the tubes running from the back of the nose to the middle ears (the *eustachian tubes*) can get blocked in hay fever. These tubes are important both as a means of equalizing air pressure on both sides of the ear drums and as a means of draining the middle ear of secretions. Failure of drainage makes infection much more likely. Such infection can be very persistent and can lead to hearing defects.

Good hearing is essential if children are to develop normal speech and realize their full mental capacity. One of the most common ways in which hearing is affected in children is by middle ear disease. This can be very insidious, for the child is quite unaware of what is happening and will never complain that he or she cannot hear. Any child who suffers for any length of time from allergic problems of this kind should have an audiogram check of the hearing.

Allergic asthma

Although hay fever is not especially common in children, you will see in Chapter 8 that one important complication of IgE-mediated allergy can be quite serious, especially in the case of children. Here is a case history that illustrates this point.

Introduction

Brook has an allergic tendency which, at first, produces only an allergic rhinitis. Part of the problem is allergy to microscopic particles of household dust. Control of these factors helps considerably but Brook still has fairly frequent attacks. At the age of nine, however, matters take a more serious turn.

Personal details

Name Brook Saunders
Age 9
Occupation Schoolgirl
Family Parents alive and well. Two brothers in good health

Medical background

Brook has had a tendency to eczema from birth but careful management of her skin has kept this under control. She started to have hay fever-like attacks when she was three years old and these have become gradually more severe. Both of Brook's parents are heavy cigarette smokers. Her mother is familiar with the problems of allergy as there is a well-marked family history of hay fever, eczema and asthma on her side, affecting two of Brook's aunts. Mrs Saunders is optimistic, however, as, in both cases, the trouble cleared up completely by early adult life. When Brook is nine, however, a new and alarming manifestation of her allergy occurs.

The first severe attack

The attack started quite unexpectedly with breathlessness, wheezing, and a dry cough. Brook complains of tightness in her chest. In a short time her breathing is increasingly difficult, and she is distressed and anxious. She can breathe in easily but wheezes loudly on expiration. The family doctor is summoned and he gives her an intravenous injection of aminophylline and arranges for her immediate admission to hospital.

The management in hospital

In hospital Brook is given a further intravenous injection of aminophylline and then a corticosteroid drug and another drug to widen the air tubes (a *bronchodilator*). She is also given oxygen by mask. After an hour or two her condition improves dramatically and she is able to breathe easily without assistance.

The doctor's comments

Next morning, the consultant has a talk with Mrs Saunders. He tells her that Brook's allergy to house dust has now developed into a severe form of asthma. The process is essentially the same but now affects the breathing tubes rather than the nose. Her IgE levels have risen substantially. This, he says, is now known to be one of the effects in children of passive smoking. Every effort must be made to prevent further attacks by removing the cause. Bed mattresses must be sealed in polythene and thoroughly vacuum-cleaned every week. And Brook should not be exposed to cigarette smoke.

He explains that asthma is not a trivial condition and that he is going to prescribe medication to be taken by inhaler. The time to stop an asthma attack is at the very beginning and attacks must not be allowed to develop. Brook must be taught to use her inhalers properly, and when to use each kind. Any indication that inhaler treatment is having a reduced effect is a danger sign that must not be ignored. Mrs Saunders is also shown how to use a peak flow meter to check how easily air can get into and out of Brook's lungs. This is to be done every day. Brook must respond to any reduction in respiratory performance by increasing the use of the inhalers.

The follow-up

Mr and Mrs Saunders succeed in giving up smoking. In a short time Brook becomes expert in the use of her inhalers. She knows which one is for routine use to block allergic attacks and which one widens her air tubes. She also knows when to use her third inhaler to control an established attack. Brook can now monitor her breathing ability with her peak flow meter and is able to suggest when a boost in treatment is required.

10
Complications

Sinusitis

The sinuses are cavities in the bone of the skull in the region around the nose. These paired cavities exist below and above the eyes (maxillary and frontal sinuses), between the nose and the eyes (ethmoidal sinuses) and immediately behind and above the nose (sphenoidal sinuses). All these sinuses are lined with the same kind of mucous membrane as the nose, and all of them communicate with the nose by narrow, tube-like openings. These allow the secretions of the mucous membranes to drain out.

When mucous membrane gets swollen, as described in Chapter 3, it is quite common for these narrow openings (which are also lined with mucous membrane) to become closed off. This is a most unfortunate thing to happen. The inflamed mucous membrane continues to oversecrete and pressure builds up in the affected sinuses causing pain that can sometimes be distressingly severe. Fortunately, allergic sinusitis tends to be less persistent and severe than sinusitis from infection, and seldom, if ever, causes fever, general upset and inflammation of the overlying skin. If it goes on too long, however, it may become indistinguishable from infective sinusitis and its allergic origin may not be suspected. Antibiotics, which are the mainstay of the treatment of infective sinusitis, are useless in treating allergic reactions. These have nothing to do with infection.

Eustachian catarrh

Some of the complications of hay fever allergy are quite unexpected. We have already briefly come across problems with the eustachian tubes but as this seems seldom to be recognized as a manifestation of allergic rhinitis it is worth taking a closer look at this unpleasant complication. Here is a case history that covers the essential facts.

Introduction

When his hearing deteriorated Joshua was convinced that his career as a speech therapist was at an end. But his problem turned out to have a simpler solution than he had supposed. An accurate diagnosis and routine treatment were all that were necessary.

Personal details

Name Joshua Engels
Age 52
Occupation Speech therapist
Family Parents alive. Father suffers from asthma. No brothers or sisters

Medical background

Joshua is a private speech therapist who specializes in helping deaf children to articulate clearly. Although his past medical history is unremarkable, he is constantly preoccupied with his health and is inclined to be a bit of a hypochondriac. So when he suddenly realizes that his hearing has changed radically, he is seriously worried. The next day he is in Harley Street anxiously explaining his symptoms to an Ear, Nose and Throat consultant.

The complaint

The most alarming thing about the change in his hearing, he explains to the doctor, is his perception of his own voice. Instead of sounding normal, it reverberates with a horrible kind of distortion in his ears. The actual loss of hearing is comparatively slight and he can make out normal conversation. But he is convinced that if he cannot assess the quality of his own voice, he will not be able to continue with his work.

The investigation

The specialist asks a few questions and Joshua agrees that he has recently been sneezing a good deal and has had unusually watery eyes. The doctor performs an audiogram which shows a slight, general reduction in the acuity of hearing. He then carries out an examination of his ear-drums, with an auriscope, and of his nose with a fine fibre optic endoscope. He also examines Joshua's throat with a head mirror and a tongue depressor and checks the entrance to his larynx with an angled mirror. When he is finished, he asks Joshua to blow his nose and check whether his ears pop. Joshua finds he cannot influence his ears by doing this.

The consultant then explains that he proposes to anaesthetize the inside of Joshua's nose and pass a fine tube called a eustachian catheter to equalize the air pressure on either side of the ear-drums. Joshua finds this unpleasant but not painful. As soon as air is blown through the catheter on both sides, Joshua realizes that his hearing is back to normal.

The diagnosis

The consultant explains that Joshua has eustachian catarrh – an inflammation of the linings of the tubes that run from the back of the nose to the middle ear. This has caused the linings of the tubes to swell and the tubes to close. The air in the middle ears has then been absorbed into the blood vessels of the mucous membrane, so that the ear-drums are forced inwards by atmospheric pressure and are no longer able to move freely. Passing a tube to let the air into the middle ear (*eustachian catheterization*) has temporarily corrected the problem.

Joshua asks what has caused the inflammation and is told that this is usually due to infection of the nose or throat. As there is no sign of this, the trouble is probably an allergy. This also fits in with the sneezing, the eye watering and the time of the year. This is an unusual symptom of hay fever but the specialist has seen several cases like this before.

The treatment

Joshua is greatly relieved to learn that his problem is not permanent. They discuss treatment. Joshua explains that he is not particularly keen to take antihistamines as he fears that this may lower his concentration. The doctor assures him that there are antihistamines that do not have this effect, but prescribes a cromoglycate nasal spray to be used as a preventive (see Chapter

7). Fortunately, this is sufficient to prevent further episodes of eustachian catarrh.

The follow-up

Joshua needs to use the spray only during the pollen seasons, and, on the whole, succeeds in avoiding ear trouble for several years. Gradually, however, his hay fever gets worse and eventually he requires more vigorous treatment. He is now using a combination of cromoglycate drops, a steroid nasal spray and carefully selected antihistamines (see Chapter 6). His doctor is considering referring him to an allergist with a view to possible desensitization treatment.

Urticaria

One of the important effects of histamine released from mast cells is the action it has on the smallest of all blood vessels – the capillaries. These vessels are very thin-walled and normally allow a certain amount of water to pass out from the blood at the high-pressure (arterial) end and in again at the low-pressure (venous) end. Histamine interferes with this effect so that much more water than usual passes out. In areas where histamine is present near the surface of the skin, therefore, there will be local, balloon-like swellings in the skin. This is called *urticaria* or *angioedema*. Urticaria is not necessarily an allergic process and it is not a direct complication of hay fever, but it is commonly an IgE problem so is much more likely to affect people who have hay fever. It may be caused by drugs such as aspirin, some food additives such as tartrazine, certain foods such as yeasts, and plant and insect stings. Mild and moderate urticaria responds well to antihistamine drugs.

Anaphylactic shock

Happily, this serious allergic effect is rare, even in hay fever sufferers. But it is commoner in these than in non-allergic people. As we have seen, histamine is very powerful stuff. When it reaches mucus gland cells and the small glands that produce a watery fluid, it causes them to secrete strongly. When it reaches the blood vessels in the lining of the nose it causes them to widen so that the whole area becomes flooded with blood. When it reaches the smooth muscles surrounding the air tubes of the lungs (*bronchioles*), it causes them to tighten so that the bronchioles are narrowed and there is difficulty in breathing. Fortunately, the action of histamine is mainly confined to the area in which it is released from the mast cells. But if large amounts are released it can get into the bloodstream and have its effect all over the body. This can be very dangerous because the effects are so widespread. A general widening of blood vessels causes a serious drop in the blood pressure, and the effects on the lungs can be devastating. This generalized effect is called anaphylactic shock and it is often fatal. You may have heard of people killed by a single bee sting. This is how it happens. The affected person must, of course, have been previously sensitized by an earlier sting and must have accumulated IgE.

People who readily produce IgE are more prone to this rare condition than others and should know about it. This is especially important if there has been a previous anaphylactic episode. It may be caused by a drug such as penicillin or aspirin, by an insect sting, by injudicious attempts at desensitization (see Chapter 7), or by any circumstance in which an allergen that can trigger off widespread histamine release is introduced into the body. Apart from the catastrophic drop in blood pressure there is an even greater danger. The soft tissues lining the larynx are especially prone to oedema and if this occurs the airway may be cut off completely. This is probably the most acute emergency of all. Anyone with a closed airway has only minutes to live.

Emergency treatment is by an injection of adrenaline and an antihistamine and, in the most severe cases, an intravenous injection of a steroid. Often an emergency opening has to be made into the windpipe in the neck as the only way of saving life. This is called a *tracheostomy*. It may sound drastic, but there are critical circumstances in which it is the only thing to do. The victim's neck is extended and a bold cut is made with a sharp knife or a razor blade vertically downwards immediately below the projection of the Adam's apple. As soon as the windpipe is opened breathing can occur and a small tube of some kind – maybe the barrel of a ball-point pen – is pushed in to keep the hole open. Many lives have been saved by this kind of crude surgery, performed on the spot.

Asthma

About ten per cent of people with hay fever or PAR develop asthma. One child in ten suffers from asthma. So, obviously, this is something you should know about. Asthma is a major subject in its own right and this book is about hay fever, so only a general outline can be given here. Like hay fever, asthma is becoming more common, and badly managed asthma can be dangerous. Unfortunately, people do sometimes die from asthma, often because no one was aware of the danger signs. Asthma is commonest in atopic people (see Chapter 2).

The air tubes leading to the lungs are called *bronchi* and they have muscle rings in their walls which, under the influence of histamine, can tighten up to cause severe narrowing of the airway. The triggers for histamine release are exactly the same as in hay fever and PAR. These are listed in Chapter 2. In general, the smaller the allergen particles, the more likely they are to get down to the lungs. Asthma can also be triggered by colds, coughs or bronchitis, or even by exercise, especially in cold weather. Emotional factors, such as stress or anxiety, may precipitate attacks.

Asthmatic attacks vary greatly in their severity and are most frequent in the early morning. The main symptoms are:

- breathlessness;
- wheezing;
- a dry cough sometimes brought on by exercise;
- a feeling of tightness in the chest.

During a severe attack, breathing becomes increasingly difficult, causing sweating, rapid heart beat, and great distress and anxiety. The sufferer cannot lie down or sleep, may be unable to speak, breathes rapidly, and wheezes loudly. In a very severe attack, the low amount of oxygen in the blood may cause blue-purple discoloration of the face, particularly the lips. This is called *cyanosis* and it is a clear sign of the severity of the attack. In addition, the skin may become pale and clammy. Such attacks may be fatal. In Britain, about 2,000 people die from asthma each year. Twice as many die from asthmatic complications.

Asthma attacks can be prevented or minimized to a large extent. First the allergen must be identified and avoided if possible (see Chapters 5 and 11). More successful in preventing attacks are drugs, such as *cromoglycate* (*cromolyn sodium*) and inhaled steroid drugs. To be effective, they must be taken several times daily from an inhaler.

Once an attack has started, a preventive drug has limited effects and a drug that relaxes and widens the airways (a bronchodilator), such as *Ventolin, Cyclocaps* or *Salbulin* (*salbutamol*), *Bricanyl* (*terbutaline*) or *Duovent* (*fenoterol*), must be used. If you are asthmatic, you must learn the proper way to administer the drug yourself with an inhaler. Most attacks of asthma either pass naturally or can be controlled by use of a bronchodilator. In some cases, however, an attack may be so severe that it fails to respond to the recommended dose of the drug. In this case, you should repeat the dose. If this has no effect, see a doctor or get yourself to hospital without delay. It is essential to understand that if, in spite of treatment, your asthma is going out of control, this is an emergency situation that requires urgent medical attention, day or night.

There is much more to be known about asthma and you should study one of the many popular books on the subject. Above all, you should, at all time, know about the state of your bronchial tubes. Ideally, you should be regularly checking, with a peak flow meter, the rates at which you breath out. You should be keeping a record of the results, and should know at what point the peak flow rate has become dangerously low.

11
Avoiding Hay Fever

Prevention is always better than cure, and in the case of allergic rhinitis this is particularly so. Avoiding contact with the allergen – once you have discovered what it is – is especially important because, as we have seen, *hay fever gets worse with repeated exposure*. The progressive increase in the amount of IgE and in the number of mast cells and basophil cells means that complications and possibly even irreversible disease become more likely.

Never be content simply to know that you have hay fever; it is essential to know precisely what the allergen is that is causing it. Only when you do know this can you intelligently plan an avoidance strategy. If you are very fortunate, you may be able to avoid the allergen altogether, and if you can do this, you might even be able to cure your hay fever. Unfortunately, it is extremely difficult to avoid allergens completely.

Keeping away from the allergen

An obvious measure is to limit your movements so as to avoid areas in which your allergen is prevalent during hay fever seasons. During these periods you can greatly help to reduce trouble by:

- staying indoors;
- keeping windows closed, even upper-floor windows in tall buildings;
- keeping car windows closed during country trips;
- observing reports of high pollen counts;
- avoiding parks and other open spaces with vegetation;
- keep away from barns, grass mowing, haymaking;
- wearing close-fitting sunglasses or even goggles;
- wearing a mask over the nose and mouth.

Unfortunately, simple masks are far from effective in keeping out tiny particles of the size of pollen grains. If you want to do this really effectively, the only way is to use a kind of spherical space helmet, sealed around the shoulders and connected by a wide tube to a portable, battery-powered filter unit on a belt. This unit can eliminate allergens. Very few people are willing to go this far. Most would feel uncomfortably conspicuous. There is another reason for discomfort. In sunny weather, when you are most likely to need such a device, the greenhouse effect leads to an unpleasant rise of temperature within the globe. You may also find the plastic mists up.

Indoors, it is possible to use electrostatic particle precipitators and high-efficiency air-conditioning systems with particle-trapping filters. These are major and expensive items, not to be confused with domestic 'ionizers'. Note, however, that while such equipment can clear tiny particles such as pollen grains, you will still be in trouble if your problem is caused by heavier particles such as house mite faecal allergens. These pass briefly into the air when mattresses, bedding etc. are disturbed and may be inhaled. But they soon settle again and are not removed by air filters.

If you suffer from straightforward hay fever, you might consider having one room – such as a bedroom – fitted with a high-efficiency particulate air filter. You can even hire equipment of this kind for use during the hay fever seasons.

Some people have found it worthwhile to go to the length of a change of residence.

What to do about mites

Many people believe that a good weekly hoovering of bedrooms is all that is necessary. Unfortunately, this is not so. A thorough vacuum clean can reduce the mite population by 70 per cent but the population will return to the previous level within a week. Mite faeces particles are highly allergenic and you need to inhale only a few to keep the symptoms going. So if you are going to try to rely on the vacuum cleaner, you will have to use it every day.

Remember also that vacuuming causes mite faeces to become airborne, so the sufferer should keep out of the room that is being cleaned.

You must also ensure that the vacuum cleaner bag has very small pores. Stout disposable paper bags are likely to be more efficient than the earlier cloth bags that have to be emptied, but neither can be relied on to prevent small particles from passing through. Particles are more likely to be trapped if the bag has already been used for a while so that the air has to pass through a thick layer of fluff and dust. You might even decide to experiment by putting some loose cotton wool in the bag.

Mites can be killed by various chemicals such as tannic acid, crotamiton or benzyl benzoate. Some people treat their carpets with these. Unfortunately, benzyl benzoate, which is a long-established treatment for another mite problem – scabies – can cause severe skin irritation and may be damaging to the eyes. You have to be rather careful you don't overdo the use of these miticide substances.

Probably the most effective measure against mites is to deprive them of the kind of habitat they like best – cotton or linen sheets, pillowslips, duvet covers and mattresses. If you examine an ordinary bedsheet with a strong hand lens you will see that the cloth contains endless convenient little spaces for these creatures to lurk in and quietly munch on, and digest, the protein skin scales you are so kindly donating. So if you enclose your mattresses and pillows in polythene or nylon bags you will make things hard for the mites. If you decide to do this, ensure that there is no possible danger of a plastic bag coming loose and causing suffocation. Frequent washing of bedding at a high temperature setting of the washing machine will also help to keep the mite population down.

Pollen seasons in different countries

If you are a hay fever sufferer you will be thoroughly familiar with the seasons during which you are affected. You have to remember, however, that if you are planning a holiday or a stay abroad, the peak pollen and other allergen seasons may differ from those you are accustomed to. Wherever you go, try to avoid areas of extensive vegetation, especially grass meadows. The general rule in the tropics is that allergens are likely to be most profuse following rainy seasons.

There are too many countries to cover comprehensively, but here is an alphabetical list of some of those likely to be of interest.

Alpine regions

This is a recommended holiday region if you suffer severely, because pollen counts are low everywhere. You may, however, encounter some grass pollen at the end of July and the beginning of August. House mites do not survive above 1,000 metres.

The Bermudas

Like other warm island regions, such as Singapore and the Seychelles, the pollen counts are low and there is little likelihood of trouble from hay fever. The high humidity, however, does greatly encourage fungal growth. If you are susceptible to fungal allergies, these islands may not be for you.

Caribbean

The pollen counts tend to be high for most of the year with a peak during November to January. Pollen counts are lowest between August and October. There may be a year-round problem from nettles with a peak during March to June.

East Africa

The best time for travel, from the point of view of hay fever only, is during the monsoon season, from mid-June to mid-September, when the atmospheric allergen content is low. This, however, can be a very uncomfortable period from other points of view. Pollen counts can be very high between September and November. The best compromise between weather and pollen is probably between mid-February and mid-June.

Egypt

In most tourist areas grass pollens peak around June, but you may encounter nettle and goosefoot (*Chenopodium*) pollens from March to November, with a peak in April. If you are a hay fever victim you would be best to plan to visit Egypt some time between December and February.

France

Along the Mediterranean coast there is a good deal of pollen at most times of the year with a peak between late May and early June. Grass pollens are worst between April and August and nettle pollens occur between late February and September. Cypress tree pollens occur in January and February, and olive tree pollens in April to July. The west coast of France, however, is a good area for hay fever sufferers, and has low pollen counts for most of the year. In Paris, hay fever sufferers are likely to have trouble throughout most of the spring and summer, March to August.

Greece

The worst of the pollen is from March to July with a peak in May and June. Both grass and tree pollens, especially from plane trees, poplars and olive trees, are prominent during this period. Tree pollens are worst in March and April. Nettle pollens can also be a problem around the same time.

India

The situation is similar to that in East Africa. India has a monsoon climate and during the rainy periods you will have no trouble with hay fever as all the atmospheric pollution is washed away. The after-effects of the rain, however, greatly encourage the growth of grasses and other plants, and pollen counts can rise very high in October and November. So the best time to travel, from a hay fever point of view, is from mid-June to mid-September.

Italy

Along the Adriatic coast and in the Po valley the main problem is from grass pollens. The grass pollen season extends from April to June with a peak in May. Tree pollens, especially from Cypress trees, will be encountered from mid-February to mid-March. Olive trees may also cause problems with pollen dispersion at the end of May and the beginning of June.

Scandinavia

Tree pollens are the main problem because of the extensive forests. In particular, you may expect trouble from birch pollens from the latter part of May until the middle of July, especially in southern Sweden and Finland. In general, allergies from tree pollens are more troublesome in the south of Scandinavia than in the north. There is also a lengthy grass pollen season from late May until about mid-August. Nettle pollen allergens are also encountered, usually worst in June.

Seychelles

See Bermudas.

Singapore

See Bermudas.

Spain and Portugal

This is not the ideal holiday region for hay fever sufferers, especially in central and southern Spain, where you may expect to encounter pollens from February to December. The worst time of the year is May and June. Things are not so bad in the Algarve and the larger inland cities, where grass pollen counts may be quite low. But watch out for pollens from plane trees in May and June. You will find olive trees in most parts of Spain and Portugal. These cause most hay fever trouble between the end of May and the end of June.

United States

The grass pollen season in most places is from May to October, usually worst in June. In Washington, DC tree pollens are worst from February to May; grass pollens from May to June; and fungal spores from July to August. Watch out for the ragweed season which, in the eastern and midwestern States, lasts from July to October. This is a potent allergen, often called 'sneeze-weed' and is the most serious offender causing hay fever in the USA. In the south, in places like Florida, tree pollens, especially cedar pollens, peak between January and March. White oak pollens peak between February and May. In Hawaii, tree pollens are most troublesome between January and April. Weed pollens are plentiful for most of the rest of the year. You might be lucky in May. Pollen calendars are available for all the States.

Glossary

This wordlist serves two functions; it provides a convenient reminder of the meanings of words you may come across while reading the book (although all technical words are, of course, defined when they first appear), and it acts as a kind of summary or recapitulation of the medical principles underlying hay fever and perennial allergic rhinitis (PAR). Cross-references to other definitions in this section are shown in **bold.**

acute Short, sharp and quickly over. Acute conditions usually start abruptly, last for a few days and then either settle or become persistent and longlasting (*chronic*). From the Latin *acutus*, sharp.

aeroallergens Airborne particles, especially tree and glass pollens, that can induce allergic responses, such as hay fever (**allergic rhinitis**) in sensitized persons.

allergen Any substance that can provoke an allergic reaction after coming in contact with the body. Allergens are examples of **antigens** – the wider group of all the substances that the body recognizes as foreign and produces antibodies against. This book is largely concerned with allergens and you can read all about them in Chapter 2.

allergic alveolitis Inflammation of the small air sacs in the lungs, usually caused by inhalation of organic dusts. There are various named types, including Bird fancier's lung, Farmer's lung, Mushroom worker's lung, baggasosis, Maltworker's lung and Maple bark disease. Allergic alveolitis is very much less common than hay fever or PAR. It is a form of pneumonia featuring wheezing, breathlessness, dry cough, fever and a feeling of illness (*malaise*).

allergic rhinitis Hay fever. The susceptibility (**atopy**) is often inherited. A specific immunoglobulin (**IgE**) coats the mast cells in the nose and air passages. When the **allergen** – grass or tree pollen etc. – reaches the mast cells it combines with the IgE and this triggers the release of histamine and other highly irritating substances from the mast cells. Allergic rhinitis is what this book is all about.

allergy An abnormal sensitivity to body contact with a foreign substance, known as an **allergen**. The commonest allergens are grass or tree pollens, dust mites and their excreta or certain metals such as nickel. The effect may take several forms, including weals (*urticaria*), dermatitis, asthma or hay fever (**allergic rhinitis**). An allergic response implies that there has been a prior contact with the allergen during which the immunological processes leading to the hypersensitivity have occurred. Susceptibility to allergy is often inherited. *See also* **allergic dermatitis** and **allergic rhinitis**.

anaphylaxis A severe form of allergic reaction most commonly provoked by drugs such as penicillin, intravenous iron or procainamide, but also brought on by allergy to foods, vaccines, insect stings or snake bites. There is always a history of a previous reaction to the **allergen**. The effects are a drop in blood pressure, local swelling of the skin (*angioedema*), narrowing of the air tubes, itching, vomiting and abdominal pain. The sooner the onset after exposure to the allergen, the more severe the reaction. Anaphylactic shock is a serious, widespread allergic attack which may cause death by airway obstruction from swelling of the lining of the voice box in the neck.

antibody A protein substance, called an immunoglobulin, produced by the B group of lymphocytes in response to the presence of an **antigen**. An appropriate B lymphocyte is selected from the existing repertoire. This then produces a clone of plasma cells – little protein factories each capable of making large numbers of specific antibodies to combat the infection. The B cells also produce memory cells. Subsequent infection with the same antigen prompts the memory cells to clone plasma cells and produce the correct antibodies without further delay. This is an important way in which infection results in subsequent immunity. Antibodies are able to neutralize antigens or render them susceptible to destruction by phagocytes in the body. Unfortunately, the production of one type of antibody does more harm than good. You can read about this in Chapter 2.

antigen Any substance that the immune system of the body can recognize as being 'foreign'. Antigens are chemical groups on the surface of viruses, bacteria, fungi, pollen grains, donor tissue from other individuals, or any other 'non-self' material. The immune system can identify antigens and produce custom-built antibodies to attack the foreign invaders that are carrying them.

antihistamine One of a group of drugs which act to prevent histamine – a powerful and highly irritant agent released in the body by mast cells – from causing its unpleasant effects on local cells and tissues. Antihistamine drugs fall into two groups – those used to relieve allergies that block H_1 receptors and act mainly on blood vessels, and those used to reduce the rate of acid production by the stomach that block H_2 receptors. The latter are not usually called antihistamines but are well known as the drugs *cimetidine* (*Tagamet*) and *ranitidine* (*Zantac*). You can read all about antihistamines in Chapter 6.

atopy An underlying allergic tendency which may show itself in a number of different ways. Atopy is associated with immunoglobulin E (**IgE**) production and is an inherited tendency caused by a gene that alters the binding sites for IgE on **mast cells**. Atopy features a proneness to asthma, hay fever and eczema (atopic dermatitis). The term was derived from the Greek *a-*, 'not' and *topos*, 'a place', on the grounds that the reaction could occur at a different site from that of contact with the causal **allergen**. This is not the case with hay fever but occurs with anaphylactic reactions. *See also* Chapter 2.

atrophic rhinitis An unpleasant condition affecting the inner lining of the nose which becomes dry and crusty and produces a foul odour. There is loss of the sense of smell and frequent nosebleeds. This is a very rare possible late complication of severe **allergic rhinitis**. There is more about nasal problems in Chapter 1.

basophil cells Granular cells, roughly similar in appearance and effect to **mast cells**, that appear in increasing numbers in people with long-term hay fever. Like mast cells, basophils can produce powerfully irritating substances, such as histamine, with unpleasant effects. In general, basophils are less important than mast cells in the hay fever and PAR reactions. You can safely assume that when mast cells are mentioned, as in Chapter 2, basophils are also likely to be involved.

B cells One of the two main classes of lymphocytes – the white cells found in the blood, lymph nodes and tissue which, with other cells, form the immune system of the body. You should really call them 'B lymphocytes' but for convenience they are usually called 'B cells'. They are the cells that actually produce the antibodies (immunoglobulins). To do so they are quickly modified so that they become very active protein factories and, in this form, they are usually called plasma cells. They are, however, still B cells. *See also* **T cells.**

cilia The microscopic hair-like processes extending from the surface of the lining cells of the nose and other parts of the respiratory system. This lining layer is called *ciliated epithelium*. The cilia move in a coordinated rhythmical lashing motion usually described as being like a wind-blown field of corn. The point of this is to carry out of the nose and air tubes particles of dust, fluff, pollen etc. that have been caught by the sticky mucus. Healthy cilia do an excellent job in helping to condition the air passing through the nose and they ensure that pollen grains do their harm for the shortest possible time.

corticosteroid hormones Natural steroid hormones secreted by the outer zone (*cortex*) of the adrenal glands. These hormones are cortisol, corticosterone, aldosterone and androsterone. The first two, or substances chemically similar to them, are commonly used as drugs to treat hay fever, PAR and allergic asthma. They are highly effective and, because they are usually taken by inhalation, are unlikely to produce any general side effects. You can read more about the steroid drugs in Chapter 7.

cromoglycate, sodium A drug used in allergies. It is said to work by stabilizing the membrane of the **mast cells** to prevent the release of histamine and other irritating substances when antibodies (**IgE**) and **allergens** (such as pollen grains) react on their surfaces. You have to use cromoglycate before the allergens arrive. *See also* Chapter 7.

food allergy Sensitivity to one or more of the substances in normal diets. True food allergy is rare – much less common than you would think from reading popular medical books. Proper scientific tests, especially double-blind trials in which neither the tester nor the person tested know what is being given, have shown that food allergy does not cause many of the disorders commonly attributed to it. Monosodium glutamate (MSG) can cause the *Chinese restaurant syndrome*. Tartrazine sensitivity is an established fact. Other additives, such as sulphur dioxide, sulphites, azo-dyes (used in most textiles) and benzoate preservatives also sometimes cause genuine allergic reactions, such as asthma. Allergy to basic foodstuffs seldom occurs. Food intolerance is fairly common but has nothing to do with allergy.

fungi A large group of spore-bearing organisms that derive their nourishment by decomposing non-living organic matter and absorbing nutrients through their surface. The spores from various fungi commonly cause hay fever. Many fungi can infect the body but, in people with healthy immune systems, infection tends to be limited to the outer layer (epidermis) of the skin and the readily accessible mucous membranes. Immune deficiency from any cause (*see* Chapter 2) allows widespread opportunistic fungus infections of all parts of the body. Malnourishment and poor living conditions predispose to deeper fungus infections following penetrating injuries to the feet and other parts.

gamma globulin A protein, one of the five classes of immunoglobulins (antibodies). Gamma globulin, or immunoglobulin G (IgG), is the most prevalent in the blood and elsewhere and provides the body's main antibody defence against infection. For this reason it is produced commercially from human plasma and used for passive protection against many infections, especially hepatitis, measles and poliomyelitis. Hay fever is concerned with a different immunoglobulin, that might be called epsilon globulin – **IgE.**

histamine A powerful hormone synthesized and stored in the granules of **mast cells** from which it is released when antibodies attached to the cells are contracted by **allergens** such as pollens. Free histamine acts on H_1 receptors to cause small blood vessels to widen (dilate) and become more permeable to protein, resulting in the effects known an allergic reactions. Histamine also acts on receptors in the stomach (H_2 receptors) to promote the secretion of acid. H_2 receptor blocker drugs, such as Zantac (ranitidine) are widely used to control acid secretion. *See also* **antihistamines** and Chapter 6.

hypersensitivity An allergic state in which more severe tissue reactions occur on a second or subsequent exposure to an **antigen** than on the first exposure. A particular group of antibodies (**IgE**) is involved in many hypersensitvity reactions. Hay fever, PAR, allergic asthma and urticaria are all hypersensitivity reactions.

hypogammaglobulinaemia Abnormally low levels of the antibody group gamma globulin in the blood. This is a feature of some kinds of immunodeficiency and can be corrected by monthly injections of gamma globulin. *See also* Chapter 2.

Ig The commonly-used abbreviation for *immunoglobulin*.

IgE Immunoglobulin class E, an antibody class concerned with immediate hypersensitivity reactions, such as hay fever (**allergic rhinitis**), PAR and allergic asthma. IgE has an affinity for cell surfaces and is commonly found on **mast cells**, to which it attaches at certain receptor sites. A gene mutation has recently been discovered that affects IgE receptor sites on mast cells in people particularly prone to hay fever. IgE is the immunoglobulin (antibody) type with which this book is concerned.

immune surveillance A constant checking process carried out by the immune system by which cells that have been invaded by viruses and those that are in the early stages of becoming cancers are detected, attacked and, fortunately, usually destroyed. Such cells put out flags (**antigens**) indicating that something is going wrong. These antigens can be recognized by immune system cells. Immune surveillance is carried out by T lymphocytes (T cells). Without it, most of us would already be dead.

immunity The ability to resist most infections or the effects of many toxic or dangerous substances. The word does not mean what it seems to mean – complete protection. Immunity is relative. It may be present from birth or acquired as a result of infections or immunization. Active immunity involves the production of one's own antibodies (*see* Chapter 2). Passive immunity is conferred by antibodies produced by another person or animal and injected or received across the placenta or in the breast milk. Passive immunity does not last as long as active immunity.

immunoglobulins Antibodies. These are protective proteins produced by B lymphocytes (B cells). There are five classes of immunoglobulins, the most prevalent being immunoglobulin G (IgG), or gamma globulin, which provides the body's main defence against bacteria, viruses and toxins. The others are **IgA, IgD, IgE, IgG** and **IgM. IgE** is the immunoglobulin of concern to hay fever sufferers.

inflammation The response of living tissue to injury. Inflammation features widening of blood vessels, with redness, heat, swelling and pain – the cardinal signs 'rubor' (redness), 'calor' (heat), 'tumour' (swelling) and 'dolor' (pain) first recorded by the 1st century Roman physician Aulus Cornelius Celsus. Inflammation is the commonest of all the disease processes. Any word ending in *-itis* refers to inflammation of the part mentioned. Inflammation involves release of substances, known as *prostaglandins*, that strongly stimulate pain nerve endings. In hay fever, prostaglandins are released from **mast cells** along with

histamine and are partly responsible for the symptoms of the disorder.

inhalers Devices for delivering medication in aerosol, vapour or powder form to the nose, bronchial tubes and lungs, especially for the treatment of hay fever, PAR and asthma. Propulsion of the drug may be by gas under pressure or by an inhaled current of air. Drugs commonly taken in this way include steroids, decongestants and cromoglycate (*see* Chapter 7).

mast cell A connective tissue cell found in large numbers in the mucous membranes and skin and in the lymphatic system. Mast cells play a central part in allergic reactions. They contain numerous large granules that are collections of powerfully irritating chemical substances such as histamine, serotonin and prostaglandins. In people with allergies, the antibody **IgE** remains attached to specific receptors on the surface of the mast cells. When the substance causing the allergy (the **allergen**) contacts the IgE, the mast cell is triggered to release these substances and the result is the range of allergic symptoms and signs. Chromoglycate can stabilize the mast cell membrane and prevent the release of the contents.

mucous membrane The lining of most of the body cavities and hollow internal organs such as the mouth, the nose, the eyelids, the intestine and the vagina. Mucous membranes contain large numbers of goblet-shaped cells that secrete mucus which keeps the surface moist and lubricated. Many mucous membranes are also ciliated (*see* **cilia**).

nasal congestion Swelling (**oedema**) of the **mucous membrane** lining the nose, usually as a result of inflammation from histamine released as an allergic response to tree or grass pollen grains or from a common cold virus infection. Nasal congestion can be relieved temporarily by decongestant drugs but these have some major disadvantages and potential dangers (*see* Chapter 10).

nasal discharge Any fluid running from the nose that is watery or has pus (*purulent*) or blood in it. Nasal discharge usually comes from the mucous membrane of the nose or sinuses but after a head injury may come from inside the skull and consist of the cerebrospinal fluid that normally bathes the brain.

nasal obstruction Interference with the free passage of air through either side of the nose from any cause. Causes of obstruction include swelling of the mucous membrane (**nasal congestion**) from hay fever or PAR, nasal polyps, foreign bodies, or, rarely, cancer of the back of the nose.

nasal septum The thin, central partition that divides the interior of the nose into two passages. The septum consists of a thin plate of bone, behind, and a thin plate of cartilage in front. Both are covered with mucous membrane. Deflection of the septum to one side (*deviated septum*) is common and usually harmless.

nitrogen oxides These are poisonous atmospheric pollutants mainly produced by the action of sunlight on the exhaust fumes from cars and other vehicles. Their relevance to hay fever and PAR is that nitrogen oxides can interfere with the action of **cilia** in the nose. As a result, pollen grains remain on the nose lining longer than they otherwise would, thus making the hay fever worse. Nitrogen oxides also cause irritation in their own right, thereby adding to the severity of the symptoms of hay fever.

oedema Excessive accumulation of fluid, mainly water, in the tissue spaces of the body. Oedema may be local, as at the site of an injury, or general. In allergic reactions local oedema, such as urticaria, is caused by the action of histamine on small blood vessels. General oedema may be caused by allergy, injury, starvation, heart failure, kidney disease, liver disease, hormonal changes in the menstrual cycle, varicose veins or poisoning. Persistent general oedema is treated with diuretic drugs to increase the outflow of urine and so remove water from the body.

otitis media Inflammation in the middle ear cavity. This usually results from spread of infection from the nose or throat by way of the eustachian tube but may arise as a result of blockage of the tube so that drainage from the middle ear is prevented. This can be caused by hay fever. In **acute** suppurative otitis media there is rapid production of pus with a pressure rise that causes the ear-drum to bulge outwards. In chronic suppurative otitis media, there is a hole (perforation) in the drum and usually a persistent discharge (*otorrhoea*). Otitis media is persistent and insidious and commonly affects children causing unsuspected deafness and educational disadvantage. All forms of otitis media respond well to expert treatment. (*See also* Chapter 8.)

phagocytes Cells of the immune system that respond to contact with foreign objects, such as bacteria, by surrounding, engulfing and digesting them. Phagocytes occur widely throughout the body wherever they are likely to be required. Some wander freely throughout the tissues. Phagocytes act most effectively if their prey has first been inactivated by attachment of **antibody**.

phagocytosis The envelopment and destruction of bacteria or other foreign bodies by phagocytes.

pollenosis A general term for the allergic responses to atmospheric pollen grains from trees, grasses, flowers or weeds.

postnasal drip An intermittent trickle of watery nasal discharge or mucus from the back of the nose into the throat. The excess secretion usually results from inflammation of the mucous membrane of the nose, as in **allergic rhinitis** or **rhinitis** from any cause.

rhinitis Inflammation of the mucous membrane lining of the nose. Rhinitis is one of the most common human complaints and is a major feature of hay fever (**allergic rhinitis**) and of the common cold. The membrane becomes swollen, so that the air flow is partly or wholly obstructed, and its glands become overactive causing excessive mucus production and a watery discharge. Vasomotor rhinitis is the result of a disturbance of the nervous control of blood vessels in the mucous membrane. Hypertrophic rhinitis, with thickening and persistent congestion of the membrane, is the result of long-term inflammation or repeated infection. Atrophic rhinitis features shrinkage and loss of the mucous membrane, with dryness, crusting and loss of the sense of smell. (*See also* Chapter 1.)

rhinorrhea Watery discharge from the nose. This is usually due to **rhinitis**, but following a head injury with a fracture of the base of the skull, a persistent drip from the nose may be due to leakage of cerebrospinal fluid from the brain cavity.

sick building syndrome A varied group of symptoms sometimes experienced by people working in a modern office building and attributed to the building. Symptoms include fatigue, headache, dryness and itching of the eyes, sore throat and dryness of the nose. No convincing explanation has been offered but some cases are undoubtedly due to allergic reactions. Ozone from photocopiers and laser printers can make matters worse by interfering with the action of **cilia**.

sinusitis Inflammation of the mucous membrane linings of one or more bone cavities (sinuses) of the face. This almost always results from infection. There is a feeling of fullness or pain in the forehead, cheeks or between the eyes, fever and general upset. Treatment may involve surgical drainage and antibiotics. (*See also* Chapter 8.)

skin tests Investigations to determine allergic sensitivity to various substances by pricking the skin with a needle through a drop of a solution of small quantities of the substance or by applying the substance under patches (patch tests).

sneezing A protective reflex initiated by irritation of the nose lining and resulting in a blast of air through the nose and mouth that may remove the cause. The vocal cords are firmly pressed together, air in the chest is compressed and the cords then suddenly separated. (*See* Chapter 1.)

spore A single-celled form of a fungus or other simple organism by which it can be spread. Spores are capable of developing into an adult. Fungal spores often become airborne and form common **allergens**, giving rise to hay fever.

steroid drugs Drugs identical or similar to the natural steroid hormones of the outer zone (cortex) of the adrenal glands. Modern synthetic steroids are often many times more powerful than the natural hormones hydrocortisone and corticosterone. (*See also* Chapter 7.)

submucous resection An operation on the nose to relieve **nasal obstruction** by removing displaced cartilage and bone from underneath the mucous membrane of a deviated central partition (septum) of the nose. This is occasionally needed in long-term cases of **allergic rhinitis** that have led to persistent blockage (*See also* Chapter 1.)

T cells The important class of immune system cells complementary to the **B cells**. T cells fall into five distinct groups, the most important of which are the *killer* T cells and the *helper* T cells. Killer cells are aggressive lymphocytes that roam the body searching for, and destroying, abnormal cells that have been invaded by viruses or have developed cancerous tendencies. Helper T cells cooperate with **B cells** in producing the right kinds of antibodies. It is the helper T cells that are destroyed in AIDS.

vernal conjunctivitis An allergic form of inflammation of the conjuctiva probably caused by contact with spring pollens. It affects mostly young boys in tropical or sub-tropical countries. You can read more about vernal conjunctivitis in Chapter 3.

Index